The Grin

The Dark Side of Depression

Jennie Dodd

chipmunkapublishing

the mental health publisher

Jennie Dodd

All rights reserved, no part of this publication may be reproduced by any means, electronic, mechanical photocopying, documentary, film or in any other format without prior written permission of the publisher.

Published by

Chipmunkapublishing

PO Box 6872

Brentwood

Essex CM13 1ZT

United Kingdom

http://www.chipmunkapublishing.com

Copyright © Jennie Dodd 2011

Edited by Kirsty Burlton

Chipmunkapublishing gratefully acknowledge the support of Arts Council England.

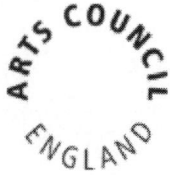

Author Biography

Jennie Dodd was born in 1950 in the picturesque market town of Shrewsbury in Shropshire. Educated at the Wakeman Grammar Technical School she developed a love of art and English literature and excelled in sport. In 1968 she entered Glamorgan College of Education where she studied advanced main physical education and subsidiary art and English for three years. She began her teaching career at the Bryntirion Comprehensive School in Bridgend, Glamorgan in 1971. She retired from teaching in 2010 and now devotes her time to writing. Jennie currently lives in Shropshire with her husband, Russell, and son, Alexander.

Jennie Dodd

Chapter 1

Beautiful Bala

As Robert drove the car that morning he felt relaxed and happy, happier in fact than he had in a long time. He sat back in the driver's seat, with just his right hand on the wheel, his left hand rested affectionately on Ruth's right hand. Every so often he would steal a glance across at his passenger and note with a feeling of warm satisfaction that she too looked comfortable and easy as if all their recent troubles had melted away. It was late Spring and a beautiful morning had dawned, the sun was high in the sky, the countryside had sprung into life and there were blossoms and leaves of all colours and shapes around them. 'I think we'll stop at Lake Bala for lunch,' he said.

'That would be nice,' Ruth replied 'Back to one of our old courting grounds!'

'Yes,' he answered smiling and remembering days gone by when they would have been on his motorbike, in their leathers, enjoying the freedom of the highway and feeling young and exhilarated, with life itself an open book before them waiting to be written.

Ruth was recovering from a nervous breakdown. She had been suffering from bouts of depression for some time and this last one had been very traumatic for them both. At one stage, her mental state had been so delicate, so fragile that Robert had almost been persuaded to have her hospitalised. Instead he had taken early retirement to be able to care for her 'round the clock.' Slowly but surely, she had improved and on seeing this improvement Robert decided that they should take a short holiday, a sight-seeing tour in North Wales. They loved climbing hills and mountains. So much so that their own home was named 'Crib y Ddysgl,' celebrating the mountain that had been their first real climb together as a young couple. They also loved visiting historic churches, manor houses and medieval castles, so North Wales was the perfect location for them for their short break.

They pulled off the road and parked in the car park of a little restaurant situated at the water's edge. It was a picture postcard setting, with hills and fields of bright green encircling a long, vivid, blue expanse of water. Llyn Tegid, otherwise known as Lake Bala, stretched over four miles in length. The blueness of the cloudless sky above them was reflected in its deep, clear waters. There was also a golden sun, high in the sky and adorning the whole landscape with light.

It was a truly glorious sun which seemed to Robert to beam down upon the Earth, especially for them. A benevolent sun that enveloped them in her warm glow and cast her magic rays far and wide to bring the world and its colours to life.

The restaurant was a black and white mock Tudor building with panoramic views across the lake. Robert chose a table by one of the many lattice windows and pulled back a chair for Ruth to sit down which would afford her the best view of the lake. 'The last time we came here,' she said, 'I was pregnant with Sean.'

'That's right,' Robert replied 'and if I remember correctly you were sick just over there,' he said pointing to a wooden bench situated under some trees to the right of the car park.

The Grim Reaper

'You've got a good memory. Well, I'll try not to do the same today,' she said laughing.

'No,' Robert agreed, 'especially since I doubt they'd give us our money back for your lunch!'

After they had eaten they strolled along the pebble beach which lined the shore hand-in-hand. 'No wonder they call this the lake of beauty,' said Ruth. A warm soft breeze caressed their happy faces and they watched enthralled as tiny sailing boats darted to and fro across the sparkling water. Gentle waves lapped at their feet creating a soothing, rhythmical sound. They listened quietly to the ebb and flow of bright water cascading over shining stones, before returning back to the lake from whence it had been born. And all the while, above their heads oak, hemlock and larch trees created a dappled, magical light through which they walked. 'I could stay here forever,' Ruth said.

'So could I,' Robert agreed. 'I've always loved this place. My aunt and uncle brought me here when I was a boy. I must have been about eight I think. Uncle Jack was a fantastic tour guide, he always knew everything there was to know about anywhere we were to visit. He frightened me actually, telling me about the local legends to do with the Lake. Its proper name is Llyn Tegid. He told me it was the largest natural lake in Wales and that below the surface, local lore would have it, the old town of Bala lies submerged. At certain times, some say, sounds from the town can still be heard, rising up out of the water. Oh and then of course,' he continued without giving Ruth time to respond, 'there was his story about Teggie.'

'What on earth is Teggie?' Ruth laughingly asked.

'Teggie,' Robert replied, 'he's the Welsh equivalent of Nessie (the Loch Ness Monster).' Ruth laughed again. 'No seriously,' said Robert, 'there have been sightings since the early 1920's. In fact I think Nessie was last caught on camera back in 1976. They say it resembles a crocodile or similar plesiosaur. The sightings were taken so seriously that a group of Japanese scientists spent several months here investigating the depths with a mini-submarine.'

'Did they find anything?' Ruth asked with interest.

'Not exactly,' Robert replied, 'but I believe they obtained a sonar trace of a very large, unidentified object, moving swiftly under the water And, of course, Llyn Tegid also has the famous - Gywniad! Before you ask, the Gywniad is a rare species of fish, left over from the last ice age.' He brought his face right up to hers and in a creepy voice said, 'it lurks some 80 feet underwater.'

'Good job,' she replied, 'if it was near the surface, you might frighten it!' They both laughed again.

By now they had walked up onto higher ground and were able to look down on the lake. The huge expanse of water lay stretched out before them. Robert heard Ruth catch her breath. 'What?' he said somewhat anxiously.

'It's just so breathtakingly beautiful,' she replied. You couldn't have a more spectacular setting, all around you high mountain peaks and hills and forests. Makes me feel glad to be alive,' she said, bringing his hand to her mouth and gently kissing his fingers one by one. 'Thank you darling,' she said, 'I'm having a wonderful day.' He wrapped his arms around her, rested his chin on her shoulder and they stood together drinking in the wonderful scenery which lay before them.

The Grim Reaper

Robert and Ruth met at the age of eighteen. He had just finished taking his 'A' levels at the boy's grammar school in the small market town of Crawley and she had done the same, taking her 'A' levels at the equivalent girl's grammar school. The chemistry between them was instant and from the moment of their meeting every hour possible was spent together. They had one particular thing in common which acted as a bond and as a result they could talk freely to each other when problems arose. They were both from unhappy homes but for very different reasons.

Chapter 2

George

Robert had been born into a working class family. His father George was a machine tool grinder at a local factory and his mother Peggy, a wages clerk at the same factory before she married. After her marriage she had been consigned to life as a housewife and later a mother. Robert's father had come from an impoverished background. He had been one of thirteen children, three of whom had died in infancy. He left school at the age of thirteen after a limited education and began his working life as a coalman. The coal was delivered by horse and cart and in all weather. It had taken its toll on his health and after a bout of pneumonia he had been advised to work indoors and had been forced to take on a particularly unpleasant job working at a chicken factory. It was poorly paid and dirty and he had hated it. Eventually, an uncle had managed to secure him an apprenticeship for a machine tool grinder at a large local munitions factory.

When at last his apprenticeship had been completed George was earning enough to consider finding a place of his own and a partner to share it with. From an early age he had never been happy at home and had received little attention from either parent. He did, however, have a kind of affection for his mother, though that relationship too was clearly tainted with bad memories – not least the fact that she had given two of her sons the same name. When George's younger brother, George Jr. was born, George was told he would have to be called Gerald from now on, since he was old enough to be grown up about a name change. As a result he grew up answering to both, but had always considered that by right his younger brother should have been the one to be renamed. He was also bitter about food or the lack of it. It seemed to him his plate was always the last one to have food put on it and often with the least amount. Memories of hunger, of going without would haunt him for the rest of his life.

He met Peggy when he went to collect his wage packet one Friday evening. They had courted, he had proposed and they were married and moved into a local council house for which they paid rent. The marriage was not a happy one although at the end they had come to depend on each other. It was love of a kind and they were comfortable together, wearing each other like one does an old pair of slippers. Robert and his sister often wondered how their parents had ever come to have children and indeed of the wisdom of that decision. Arguments were rife in the household and often over Peggy's reluctance to provide George's conjugal rights. He had a most peculiar attitude towards sex and women and often quoted his mother who believed that, 'There would be no bad men in the world if there were no bad women.' If a love scene or even a kiss was shown on television, he would storm over to the set and change channels, muttering loudly in disgust about how to display a naked body was a cardinal sin. Sometimes the television would be switched off altogether. His children never knew what it was to have an affectionate hug or kiss from their father. Being smacked, however, was a common occurrence, although in fairness to Gerald often with justification. Unhappy homes with parents at loggerheads often make for naughty children.

Arguments were even more common over his perceived opinion of her preference to give love and attention to her children rather than to him. George had yearned for love and attention throughout his childhood and he wanted his wife all to himself. Peggy had to be very careful with regards to Robert in particular. George was inordinately jealous of Robert and on several occasions she had been accused of sleeping with her own son. It seemed to both children that George resented their superior education, even though there were times when he was clearly proud. There was genuine family pleasure when they both passed the 11+ exam and went to the local grammar school and celebration when anticipated 'O' level and 'A' level exam results were achieved and university places secured. But for most of the time it was a family at war and as Robert got older the division between himself and his father in particular became more and more apparent. Physical fights had become the inevitable conclusion to arguments which could blow up in an instant and with real punches thrown. George, by now riddled with arthritis, often came off worse in these father and son battles that ended with Robert running off and not returning for hours. The whole family would be in turmoil. Tears and retribution were the order of so many bedtimes.

Perhaps the most common cause of friction within the family was food. George seemed almost to count the number of peas or potatoes on his plate, compare the size of his pork chop or portion of tuna to others around him at the dinner table. He even noted whose cup of tea was poured first! Even on the rare blue moon occasions when the family ate out, often the meal would be spoiled because he would get annoyed with the waitress for serving him last or giving him the smallest portion. There were few family outings as George believed a woman's place was in the home and so they survived on his very modest income. At George's factory, night shift workers earned slightly more than the day shift, hence George worked nights. The children had to be quiet during the day for George to sleep. Peggy would often feel the need to stop, what to them, had been enjoyable if noisy play. In the evenings, as they did their homework on the table in the living room, George would join them to eat his supper, before leaving for work. He was inevitably in an ill temper and the children were always glad when George and his pushbike, set off for the factory. In spite of George working nights, the family scrimped and scraped for money all through Robert's childhood. They remained in their 3 bed-roomed council house and aspirations of home ownership, holidays abroad, a family car or telephone, taken for granted by so many, were well beyond their reach. But, their low socio-economic status inspired Robert to work hard. He was clever and a university degree and a professional career would be his way out of poverty. He could not wait to get away from home.

Chapter 3

Janet

Shortly after leaving university, Robert and Ruth were married and happily set up their first home. Robert began working for a building company as a project's manager and Ruth had found work with a local bank. Ruth, on the other hand, felt she had no home to get away from. Her parents divorced shortly after her eighteenth birthday. Her mother Janet moved out of the family home into a small terraced house in Arlington, which at the time was a particularly deprived area of Crawley. She had been devastated by the breakup of her marriage and her health soon began to deteriorate. In February 1974 she was diagnosed with cancer. She went into hospital for what should have been a simple operation to remove gall stones. But, during the operation the doctors discovered a large tumour affecting her liver and pancreas. When Ruth and Robert called at the hospital that evening they were given the bad news. The doctor informed them that Janet had only weeks to live. The cancer was very advanced and the only medical help which could now be given would be in the form of pain relief. There was no cure. 'She is worrying about you,' the doctor said, 'hence we have not as yet told her the truth about her condition. We felt that ought to be your decision. Do you wish us to tell her?'

Almost without thinking, Ruth shook her head from side to side. 'No, no,' she said with a voice stricken with grief, 'that would spoil what little time she has left.'

Once Janet recovered from her operation she was taken to live with Robert and Ruth to recuperate. She was an emaciated figure of her former self but her demise was

The Grim Reaper

to be painful and slow. Ruth, heavily pregnant, tended to her bedridden mother's needs. Her only help came from a day nurse, who called every day between two o'clock and four o'clock and Robert, of course, did his best to help in the evenings after work. As each day passed more morphine was administered to Janet as her condition worsened. One Sunday, four weeks after her release from hospital, Ruth phoned for an ambulance. She had been sitting with her mother all night. Janet's pain had been unbearable and the morphine had done little to alleviate her suffering. Ruth could not bear to see Janet in so much pain and felt powerless to help. 'She needs to be in hospital now,' she had said to Robert, 'At least there they ought to be able to ease her suffering.' Ruth travelled with Janet in the ambulance. Janet was given a private room at the hospital and Ruth stayed with her all day. Ruth regretted her decision to keep the truth about her mother's cancer from her. Janet was dying. She was suffering and had little time left. Only a vain hope remained.

To make matters worse, every conversation between mother and daughter was now false and meaningless. Janet had always wanted to visit Italy, to see Florence, Venice and Rome. Ruth found herself making ridiculous promises, that when Janet was well they would all go on holiday together. They would visit the Coliseum, Vatican City, the Sistine Chapel and ride on a gondola under the Bridge of Sighs. She wanted to tell her mother how much she loved her, to comfort her, but to do so would have given away the truth and so real words, genuine words were never spoken. The morning after Janet returned to hospital, the staff nurse looking after Janet telephoned Ruth shortly after 8.a.m., 'Your mother has been asking for you, she is in a lot of pain. How quickly can you get here?'

When Ruth arrived less than twenty minutes later, the injection had already been given. Janet was asleep and Ruth sat by her bedside, holding her mother's hand. Janet looked little more than a skeleton, her face was hollow and her skin jaundiced. Her breathing was laboured and shallow. Even as heavily drugged as Janet was, Ruth could hear a low groan from her mother as if still in pain and the hand she was holding would tense briefly and Ruth would grip it more tightly, wanting Janet to know that she was there, that she was not alone. Janet had a particular cologne she liked with her (4 7 11) and Ruth would dampen some cotton wool with it and gently wipe her mother's brow, talking softly to her all the while.

Ruth could not bear to see her mother suffering so and she began to pray. 'Please come and take her. Please let her die and end her suffering.' Her prayer was answered. A little after midday, Janet took her last breath. Ruth heard a long almost rattling sound as Janet exhaled for the last time. Then there was silence. Ruth knew instinctively that her mother had died. She leant over and kissed Janet on the forehead and experienced the oddest sensation. She felt as if she had kissed an empty vessel. In a way it served to reaffirm her Christian faith. Her mother was no longer there, her spirit had flown and only her mortal remains, her body lay on the hospital bed. She wanted to close the open, staring eyes, which had nothing like a look of peace about them, but could not. She sank back in the chair and putting her head in her hands closed her eyes instead. Robert arrived only minutes later. It would be the first time that he recognised he had a special connection, almost a telepathic bond with his wife. He had been driving back to his office, when he had heard Ruth praying and had known immediately that Janet was close to death. He had driven straight to the hospital. He

The Grim Reaper

told the surprised staff nurse that Janet was dead. They entered the small private room together and the nurse finally, gently closed Janet's unseeing eyes.

Ruth was very low in spirit. She regretted not being honest with Janet about her illness and she couldn't put the awful image of her mother's emaciated, yellow face out of her mind. A friend advised that she go and see her mother lying at rest in the funeral parlour. 'They make them look really pretty,' she said, 'it will help you stop remembering her suffering and you'll be able to see her more like she was before her illness.' Robert advised against it and so Ruth waited her moment and went alone. Shortly after Robert left for work one morning, Ruth telephoned the funeral parlour to arrange a visitation later that day. When she arrived she was shown into one of the gathering rooms where her mother was lying at rest in an open casket. The room was dimly lit with the open coffin at its centre. It took some time before Ruth could make her legs take the necessary steps towards the casket. She fumbled in her hand bag for the Blue Grass perfume, her mother's favourite, that she had brought with her. She approached the casket with the perfume in her hand and looked down upon a face she didn't recognise.

Her mother had hardly ever worn make up in life. A tiny amount of pale pink lipstick was all Ruth could ever remember Janet wearing. This face wore a garish thick red lipstick. The skin was plastered in a thick powder, so much so that Janet's complexion was almost as white as alabaster and the eyes were heavily shadowed with a bright blue liner. Ruth felt as if she were in some horrid, grotesque, macabre pantomime. Janet's body had been dressed in a pale blue nylon burial garment. Nylon was a material Janet had always hated in life and she would never wear it next to her skin. Ruth felt somehow outraged, shocked and far from alleviating the terrible image of her mother in death at the hospital, she now felt worse. Ruth knew that Janet would have hated how she had been made to look, the awful, gaudy make-up, the nylon robe and unable now to change any of it, Ruth's sadness and remorse increased tenfold. The perfume was returned to her handbag with trembling hands. Ruth couldn't remember leaving the Funeral Director's. She found herself walking along the river bank in the town park, the Riverside, where she and Robert had first met. She was standing on the suspension bridge when Robert approached. He said nothing, simply took her hand in his and walked her over the bridge to the Waterside Inn car park, where he had parked his car. He didn't need to ask her anything, once again he had seen it all in his mind's eye and he knew exactly how desolated by grief, his wife was feeling.

Janet was buried on a cold, damp day in the November. Keith helped Ruth to arrange the funeral but there was now an insurmountable gulf between father and daughter. They hardly conversed during the entire day. Other relatives noticed the coldness between them. Ruth blamed Keith's treatment of Janet for her mother's early demise. The sadness was made even more heartbreaking for Ruth, in that her mother had died during Ruth's first pregnancy. Janet missed out on welcoming her one and only grandson into the world by just two months. Ruth's first bout of depression followed Sean's birth. She had a particularly tough labour which lasted for three days. Sean had been a forceps delivery and Robert who was present throughout the labour and the birth vowed he would never put his wife through that again. Sean was their only child.

Chapter 4

Parenthood

It had been on the occasion of Sean's birth when Robert again experienced a kind of mental telepathy with his wife. Ruth had been at the hairdressers when the first labour pain struck. Robert had been at his desk. He felt a sharp pain in his abdomen and in his mind's eye pictured Ruth doubled over, in the hairdresser's chair. He was on his way to the maternity hospital even before Ruth managed to call him, to say she had gone into labour. There were times during the birth when masculine pride steeled Robert's resolve not to ask for gas or air for himself. He knew exactly what Ruth was going through because he was feeling her pain. From the moment of Sean's birth however, Robert had been a besotted father. Declining the offer of cutting the umbilical cord, he had only minutes later shed real tears of joy, when given his baby son to hold for the first time. 'Look at him Ruth, look at him. Isn't he beautiful, just so beautiful?'

Robert had been in the habit of speaking to Ruth's heavily pregnant tummy for several months. This usually happened, either first thing in the morning before he got up for work or most particularly, last thing at night when they went to bed. In fact Ruth had often complained that after Robert's little bedtime chats the baby would start doing cartwheels in the womb, instead of sleeping peacefully.

As Robert held his baby son in his arms he spoke soothingly to him, 'Don't cry my little boy, all over now. Daddy's got you, Daddy's got you.' As if instantly recognising his father's voice, baby Sean, who had been crying, stopped.

Even the midwife exclaimed, 'well I never! Somebody knows Daddy's voice by the looks of it.' Even in her discomfort Ruth shed tears of happiness as she watched her husband's absolute joy at the birth of their son. She saw how gently he cradled the tiny infant in his arms and with a feeling of inexplicable contentment she felt herself fall in love with Robert all over again.

It had been such a difficult and traumatic delivery for Ruth that she found the first few weeks of motherhood very testing to say the least. Her body was incredibly sore, every movement was painful and sitting down was not easy, even with the ring she had been given. They intended for Sean to be breast fed, but due to Ruth's poor physical condition, they decided bottle feeding would be a better alternative. Robert took to this like a duck to water. He was a natural at parenting, preparing and sterilising bottles, feeding, winding and changing nappies with consummate ease. He took everything in his stride as if he had been doing it all his life. Ruth was also nurtured. He cooked wholesome meals for them both and refused for her to do any house work. A system for feeding Sean was devised and whilst Ruth insisted on doing the night feeds during the week, Robert took over on Friday and Saturday to give her two whole nights of sleep. Her body healed quickly and Sean thrived. Robert and Ruth soon found themselves entering into a period of matrimonial life which was extremely happy. A happiness Robert felt was almost overwhelming at times, having as he had now, two loves which knew no boundaries. Firstly the love of his beautiful wife and secondly, his now most precious newborn baby son.

The Grim Reaper

Baby Sean did not change his parent's world; he merely joined them in theirs. Two on a bike, became three on a bike with side-car. Two mountain climbers scaling the heights of Snowdon, became two plus baby carrier. A carrier not only safely and warmly transporting baby Weston to the summit, but also carefully packed with the inordinate amount of baby gear required for a successful expedition, from nappies, to baby wipes, to scented sanitation-bags, to bottles, jars of baby food, spoons, changes of clothes and more besides. As soon as a new mountain baby product came on the market it was in Sean's growing wardrobe and Robert would proudly dress his little son for every outing. Ruth often noticed how Robert would also disappear from the lounge when watching television in an evening. She always knew where to find him. He would be standing over Sean's cot watching his precious son sleep. 'I just cannot get over how beautiful he is! He's got his father's striking good looks of course.' He would say with a wry smile.

'What's he got of me then?' Ruth would ask with interest.

'Well, he's small at the moment and he smiles a lot, especially when he's got wind!' Robert would answer teasingly, before sweeping her off her feet and carrying her through to their bedroom.

Chapter 5

Keith

Ruth's father was delighted at the arrival of his grandson. Keith was an outgoing man, dark-haired and attractive in his youth, full of confidence but a renowned flirt and womaniser. In 1965 he had met an attractive 40 year-old divorcee with whom he had had an affair and she had been the reason he asked Janet for a divorce. Janet had always known that Keith had not been faithful to her through the years that they had been married but he had always come back. Janet had on a number of occasions turned a blind eye and let the affairs run their course, always expecting them to run out of steam and trusting that Keith would eventually return to her. The affair lasted less than two years but Keith did not return to Janet. Their divorce by this time was absolute anyway and he was pleased to have his freedom back again.

He was an active man, had a good social life, played golf regularly and was almost a nightly visitor to his local pub in the village of Kildale where he lived and was captain of the pub's Pool team. His wicked sense of humour and quick wit made him a favourite with the regulars. A builder by trade and built the large four bed-roomed bungalow in which he now lived himself. His career had been successful and left him with substantial money and property. He loved Sean and spent many hours with him. Ruth found herself slowly able to forgive the way that he had treated her mother. She knew how lucky she was to have found her kindred spirit in Robert and that their love was so different to that of her parent's. She was truly blessed with a match made in heaven and how therefore could

The Grim Reaper

she justify carrying a grudge against her father, when clearly he had been so less fortunate than she, in his choice of a life partner.

Twenty years passed in the blink of an eye. It was Sean's 21st party in January and all the extended family had gathered. Keith arrived with an unexpected guest. She was introduced as Lydia. They had been at school together and had been childhood sweethearts. During the Second World War circumstances had separated them and they had lost touch. Keith went to fight and Lydia's family moved out of the area. Over forty years later and quite by chance, the pair bumped into each other whilst shopping in Crawley's town centre. They went for a cup of coffee together and realised that the old feelings they once had for each other were still there. Lydia was a widow. Her husband had died three years earlier. She was now living on her own in a small council flat in the Arlington area of Crawley - ironically, just a stone's throw from the house Janet had moved into after her split from Keith. Lydia had four children, three married daughters and a son and eleven grandchildren.

Just four months later, on May 4th, Lydia and Keith were married at the registry office in Crawley. Ruth had done all she could to deter Keith from marrying so quickly, but to no avail. Keith was determined, he pointed out that Lydia had been his first true love. He was convinced that she had always been the one for him the one he should have married had not the war separated them. Lydia to him was like Robert was to her. Ruth could not argue and found herself assisting with the preparations often, she felt, to the annoyance of Lydia and her army of a family.

Keith and Lydia enjoyed an all too brief honeymoon period. At first Ruth continued to visit her father on a regular basis as she had always done. Gradually as the weeks passed she began to feel more and more unwelcome. Whenever she visited with Sean they received a less than cordial reception from Lydia and her family. It seemed that Keith had little time now for his grandson and unlike before they were never left alone together. Lydia made her displeasure in their visits quite clear in the lack of interest she showed in Sean, not even bothering to listen to him when he had something to say and interrupting him at times, especially if he was trying to converse with his grandfather. Lydia neither looked at, nor smiled nor spoke to Ruth or Sean. Her body language spoke volumes, the crossed arms and legs when sitting in their presence and the need to find the chair positioned as far away as possible from them. Ruth received the silent message loud and clear. Lydia was now Keith's wife and they had no business being there. As far as she was concerned, neither Ruth nor Sean were to be given any consideration. Only her family mattered now and if she had anything to do with it Keith would follow in her lead. Then Lydia's eldest daughter separated from her husband and she and her three children moved in with Lydia and Keith. Even before their first Christmas, having only been married for six months, it was obvious that Keith had made a big mistake. Rows began with Lydia, usually ending with Keith packing a suitcase and arriving on Ruth's doorstep, seeking sanctuary. He would often stay for days at a time.

After one such occasion in the April of their first year of marriage, he returned home to his bungalow after a two week separation, to find that Lydia had changed the locks. All his clothes had been placed in black bin liners and left in the wood store for him to collect. After months of wrangling, with solicitors playing ping pong with letter after letter passing to and fro between the estranged

The Grim Reaper

couple, Keith was finally allowed back into his own home. Lydia lodged an official complaint with the police, stating that Keith had a dreadful temper and could be violent towards her as well as himself. Keith, meanwhile, had been advised by his solicitor to stay in his home. Keith was told that possession was nine-tenths of the law and if he moved out of the property, he would virtually be handing the bungalow over to Lydia. The atmosphere in the house was unbearable, but Keith was determined to battle it out. He continued to tell Lydia that he had made a terrible mistake and it would be best if they separated. But Lydia was refusing a legal separation or to consider divorce. Robert and Ruth suspected that she now had the type of home she had always wanted and was not going to let go easily. Keith began to despair of ever getting her out.

Then another bombshell fell. Lydia's youngest son decided to follow in his sister's footsteps and split up from his girlfriend. Lydia, against Keith's wishes, gave her consent and he also moved into the bungalow. Less than a week later the police were called to the house. There had been a fight. Keith had a nasty head wound, an enormous black eye and several broken ribs. Furniture, windows and ornaments had been smashed. Due to the complaint the police had on record, which Lydia made before, and because of his age and his injuries, they insisted Keith went to hospital. Lydia complained to the Authorities again claiming that Keith's unreasonable behaviour and violent temper was putting her and her family at risk.

Chapter 6

The darkness begins

Three days later Keith telephoned Ruth from the hospital. He asked her to collect him as soon as possible and sounded anxious and worried. 'I feel as if there is something going on behind the scenes, which the nurses are not making me a party to. A different doctor came to see me this morning and was asking me all kinds of questions about my mental state. I told him the truth about Lydia. She is doing my head in after all and that I just want her out of my life and my own home back. He kept taking notes as we were talking. It made me feel really uncomfortable. I need to get out of here, Ruth, please be as quick as you can in coming. The sooner I'm away from here the better.'

By the time Robert and Ruth had arrived at Crawley hospital it was too late. Keith had already been taken off the ward by two men dressed in white coats. Against his wishes he had been removed from Crawley Hospital and transported to Claymore Hospital, an institute for the mentally ill. Now it was Ruth's turn to be angry and upset. She spoke to the staff nurse on the ward. 'I don't understand what's gone on,' she said. 'I've just come to collect my father at his request and I'm told he's already gone.' The staff nurse explained that Mrs Evans requested that her husband be sectioned because of fears over his mental state. 'What fears?' Ruth demanded.

'All I know is that Mr Evans has apparently threatened to do himself harm, has also threatened violence to his wife and over recent weeks has been in the habit of driving his car at perilous speeds when not in control of

The Grim Reaper

his emotions. Mrs Evans felt he had therefore been a real danger to himself and others on the roads. The doctor spoke to your father this morning and he felt there was justified cause for concern.'

'There is nothing wrong with my father, other than that fact that he's made a terrible mistake in marrying that awful woman,' Ruth returned with exasperation.

'Well, I'm sorry Mrs Weston,' the staff nurse went on, 'but I'm not here to be a marriage guidance counsellor. I was given an instruction to prepare Mr Evans to be taken to Claymore Hospital on bona fide medical grounds. I'm afraid you'll have to take the matter up with them. Now if you'll excuse me, I have my work to be getting on with.'

Ruth was horrified. 'What does all this section business mean?' she said to Robert as they returned to the car.

'I don't honestly know,' he replied. 'We'll need to ask the relevant questions when we get to Claymore hospital and find out what we can do to help your father out of this awful situation. I don't like the sound of this Ruth. I don't like the sound of it at all!' Unfortunately, Keith did himself no favours neither on his departure from Crawley hospital nor on his arrival at Claymore and in a way played right into the hands of the Authorities. He physically fought with the two men sent to collect him and was forcibly dragged along the corridor in a restraining jacket. He was angry and abusive to the doctors and the nursing staff on arrival at Claymore and demanded to be released and allowed home. His behaviour was such that within half an hour of his being taken up on to the ward, he had been heavily sedated. When Ruth and Robert arrived he was too heavily drugged even to converse with them. They demanded to see the doctor in charge of his case.

Finally, after a lengthy wait the doctor was able to see them. 'We don't understand what he's doing here,' Robert said. 'He's not mentally ill. He's just upset at being trapped into a rushed and now very unhappy marriage.'

'Mrs Evans believes his feelings towards her have changed because of his illness and she wants him well again. This is why she has asked for the section order to be carried out,' the doctor replied.

'What exactly does being sectioned mean?' Ruth asked, trembling.

'Well, Mrs Evans has gained legal permission to have Mr Evans, your father, receive compulsory assessment,' answered the doctor, 'and if necessary, treatment for any mental health problems which I and my staff diagnose.'

'I'd much rather just take him home with us,' Ruth replied.

'I'm afraid it's not quite as simple as that,' the doctor continued, 'Mr Evans is showing classic symptoms of depression. I went to speak with him this morning in Crawley hospital to make my assessment and I am afraid to say the signs of severe depression are there. Unless he receives help, I would anticipate matters will only worsen.'

'What signs exactly?' asked Robert.

'He appears to me to be very agitated, irritable and expressed an opinion that he was in a hopeless situation. I asked him if he had contemplated or threatened to take his life. He confirmed in his own words that he had warned Mrs Evans that if she didn't leave him, he might kill himself. You must see my concerns surely?' the doctor asked gravely.

'But he's just saying that because he wants her out and she is refusing to move,' Ruth blurted out indignantly. 'My dad is not ill. He does not need to be here!'

'In that case his stay should be of short duration. Now if you will excuse me I have patients to attend to.' The doctor rose from his chair, stone-faced and with a gesture of his hand invited then both to leave.

They went back onto the ward but Keith was still heavily sedated. The ward smelt of human sweat and urine and some of the patients were frightening in their aspect to Ruth. The windows were so high up all you could see were dark, brooding clouds moving rapidly across a cold grey sky. The ward seemed equally dark, sinister and unfriendly. 'Let's get out of here,' said Ruth shivering, 'there's nothing more we can do today.' When they got home Ruth rang Keith's old number. Eventually Lydia answered but as soon as she realised Ruth was on the other end, the phone went dead. The next day they decided to visit her in person, but again, as soon as Lydia opened the door and saw Ruth and Robert standing outside, the door was slammed shut. Robert had resisted the urge to break it down.

Chapter 7

Locked away

Crawley hospital first opened in 1840 as the County and Borough Lunatic Asylum. Robert hadn't actually told Ruth, but he had been to Claymore once before and had unpleasant memories of the place. Only a couple of years before, his company had been hired by the hospital to refurbish some of the wards in the older, Victorian part of the building. He particularly disliked seeing the locked wards and had been surprised by his reaction to being inside them. Robert was not normally known for being susceptible to the paranormal, in fact just the opposite, but he really felt an evil presence and was always glad when it was time to leave. The locked secure wards were on the top floor and they were dreadful to behold and reminded Robert more of a prison than a hospital. The rooms with their iron-barred walls and windows were a grim reminder of life in a lunatic asylum. Robert found himself blotting out visions of twisted, maniacal faces from his mind.

Ruth felt as if her father might as well have been in a locked ward. Lydia was his next of kin and therefore her word and that of the doctors at the hospital was law. They even struggled to get permission to take him off the ward for an afternoon out, let alone, get him released altogether. The treatment he received began to take an irreversible toll on his mind and his body. Ruth felt powerless. It was as if she was paralysed and as such, unable to give Keith the support he so badly needed. She felt useless and could only stand by and watch his awful treatment continue. His so-called medication and psychiatric help increased, including forced electro shock therapy and Ruth could do nothing

The Grim Reaper

to stop it. As a result, Keith's detention and suffering continued unabated. Days turned into weeks and weeks into months with little sign that he would ever be released. Ruth visited almost every day and watched his slow decline. He was fed a daily cocktail of drugs and if he was difficult in his behaviour towards the nursing staff or if he refused medication or became angry, electro shock therapy was administered against his will. After these treatments Ruth noticed how it was sometimes impossible to engage Keith in a meaningful conversation, he often appeared disorientated and confused. At such times she would try to remind him of happier days but his memory too had clearly been affected and he often had no recollection of events which in previous times they would have laughed about or held fond memories of together.

Sometimes when Ruth visited, Keith was so heavily drugged she could get no response from him at all. She hated visiting, even when she could at least converse with him, the ward was noisy and often fraught with tension. Many of the patients were frightening, most had one kind of behavioural disorder or another and often she would be approached and feel threatened, exposed and embarrassed. Worst of all were the times when Keith lost control of his own bodily functions. These often coincided with the electric shock treatments, the after math of which would leave Keith incontinent. He would often wet himself and despite her pleas to nursing staff to help clean him up and change his clothes Keith could wait for hours before being attended to. Ruth and Robert began to seek legal advice. Keith was now so ill it seemed to Ruth that he might never come out. Lydia, however, remained his next of kin and in that terrible circumstance, they were powerless to help him. Lydia was more than happy for him to remain where he was. Lydia had also taken over control of Keith's finances.

Deemed as mentally unfit she was given power of attorney and all his bank accounts and the deeds to the bungalow were now in her name. Keith was left with nothing. Three years later Keith was released and in all that time, Lydia had not visited once.

Keith was released into sheltered accommodation. He was given a tiny bedsit in a warden run hostel which housed other men with similar histories of mental health problems. Keith lived on weekly benefits and Ruth, Robert and Sean did what they could to make him as comfortable as possible. He never complained, Lydia, his bungalow, his life savings were never mentioned. He had the electro shock therapy to thank for that. It was there that he ended his days and once again in the month of November, Ruth was to lay her final parent to rest.

Ruth had been baking a fruit cake to take to Keith when the phone call from the hostel came through, to say that Keith had died peacefully in his sleep during the night. His body had been taken to the mortuary at Crawley hospital. When Ruth put the phone down her hands were shaking uncontrollably. Her legs had turned to jelly and she felt numb and nauseous. She grasped a kitchen chair and sat down. 'Robert, I must phone Robert,' she thought to herself. 'He'll know what to do.'

Just as she was about to pick up the receiver to telephone Robert's office, the phone rang. 'What's happened? She heard Robert's voice ask. 'Is it Keith?'

Chapter 8

Abandoned

Unlike Janet's funeral, the day was bright and sunny. Ruth looked pale and drawn and as the coffin was lowered into the ground she cried inconsolably. Robert and Sean had their arms around her but could give little if any comfort. From that day on the bouts of depression occurred more frequently and lasted longer. Robert kept Ruth's problems hidden from friends and family. Ruth would sometimes try to explain to Robert why she felt so unhappy. 'I know I have you and that we love each other deeply, but losing Mum the way I did and now Dad in that awful manner, I feel alone in the world, abandoned. I feel so guilty about praying for mum to die. I should have been asking God for a miracle to make her well again, not for death to come and take her. Thou shall not lie! Why did I decide not to tell her the truth? Had I been honest I could have comforted her, helped her through. Instead those last few weeks were agony for both of us. I did that Robert, it was my fault.'

'You acted out of love,' he said, trying to comfort her.

'The worst part is that Dad was lost to me months and months ago,' she continued. 'Just like Mum, I cannot remember the last meaningful conversation we had. He was so damaged at the end I couldn't even make him understand that I loved him. The man who came out of that hospital was a stranger to me. My dad had always been so full of life, funny, smart, loving, affectionate. He loved a good joke. You remember how quick witted he was, always had that immediate one line come back.' Robert smiled and nodded his head. 'The man we buried was nothing more than a shell of the man he had been. His personality had been destroyed, his lust for life had vanished and his energy totally obliterated. When we used to visit him at the shelter it was as if he was just an empty vessel, nothing of my dad had survived. I can't forgive the hospital and I'll never forgive Lydia. It's not like me to harbour evil thoughts but I hope she and that doctor rot in hell. Forgive me,' she said with tears streaming down her face.

'There's nothing to forgive,' he would say and 'Sean and I will never stop loving you.' For so many people mental illness still has a dreadful stigma attached to it and Robert wanted to keep Ruth's problems private, hoping upon hope that she would recover and be well again.

The weeks went by and Ruth seemed on a roller coaster of mood swings. Sometimes she would appear almost back to her old self and then at others Robert would despair of their life ever getting back to normal. Ruth had been particularly unhappy for several days and Robert had done his best to get home early from work. He hated leaving her when she was in her blackest moods and was beginning to wonder how long he could go on working full time. On this particular morning Robert had been relieved to find Ruth in a better frame of mind. They had eaten breakfast together and Smokey, their Persian cat, had been in an affectionate mood. She had jumped up on to Ruth's lap and had proceeded to lick Ruth's face for some time, purring loudly. 'Oh Robert,' Ruth had remarked, 'Phew! Her breath stinks of cat food.' They had both laughed. Robert kissed his wife goodbye on the front doorstep and left for work.

'I would have kissed you too,' he called back to Smokey as he walked down the drive to his car, 'but I've been pre-warned about your halitosis! I'll be back as soon as I can,' was his parting comment.

Chapter 9

Ruth's decline

Robert had an incredibly busy day at work. The job he was managing was not going well. His company had won a tender to build a new IT suite at a large 6th form college in Worcester. So far as Robert was concerned the job had been priced far too low. He had warned his bosses, but as always his advice had fallen on deaf ears. The project was already running well over budget and to save on costs, Robert was forced to employ sub-contractors rather than use company staff. The head teacher of the college had telephoned Robert that morning, to say that he had received a complaint regarding one of the workmen, who had apparently behaved improperly with one of the 6th form girls. The college were considering calling in the police to investigate.

Robert requested and was granted, permission to speak to the young workman first, before any action was taken and drove immediately to the college. On arrival, other problems were waiting to greet him. His workmen were standing around idle. Equipment which had been ordered had not arrived. It was proving to be a difficult and demanding day. Fortunately, after lengthy discussions with the young workman accused of indecent behaviour, Robert persuaded the head teacher not to press charges. On the information Robert had been able to give, the girl was interviewed again. She confessed that her original claims had been prefabricated. In fact, it appeared she had been the one to make inappropriate advances and when rejected, had vindictively determined to cause the young man trouble.

Robert was glad when the day drew to an end and he was on his way home. He felt exhausted and once again he found himself questioning how long he could go on fulfilling the demands of such a responsible job and still find sufficient time to help nurse his troubled wife back to health. He was travelling along the motorway, when he noticed a sign pointing out that he was coming up to a service area. The day had been so fraught that he had not had time for any lunch, so he decided to pull off the motorway and take a short stop for a coffee and a sandwich. He moved in to the left lane. The services were less than a mile off. He began to slow down and as he did so he noticed a woman sprinting along the hard shoulder just ahead of him. As he drew level he recognised her immediately. It was Ruth. She looked terrified and was running as if the devil himself was chasing her. He indicated left and pulled onto the hard shoulder. When he stepped out of the car, he found himself alone at the road side, there was nobody there. Robert knew instinctively that something was wrong. He got back into the car and drove home without delay. It was all he could do to stay within the speed limit.

Robert pulled the car up onto the drive. He could see lights on in the lounge and the kitchen and began to relax. Ruth would have telephoned him had something been wrong. He'd been feeling tired and hungry on the motorway and had allowed his imagination to run away with him. 'There must be a simple explanation,' he told himself. 'I've certainly had enough drama for one day.' He turned the key in the lock and entered into the front hallway. He was feeling ravenous and was looking forward to sitting down with Ruth and enjoying a good supper together. Just then he realised something was missing. Tea was never exactly on the table when he got home, but he could usually smell something

The Grim Reaper

cooking. He could smell the lavender air freshener, but nothing else. 'I'm home,' he called as he entered the kitchen. There was no sign of Ruth, the table had not been laid and no food had been prepared. Two bouquets of flowers were standing stems down in a dry sink. Robert's anxiety returned.

He stood still and listened. He could feel Ruth was near, but very frightened. 'Ruth, I'm home,' he began calling, trying not to sound alarmed. He moved back into the hallway and looked at the door of the cupboard under the stairs. In his mind he pictured Ruth crouched at the back with a raised knife in her right hand. 'Ruth, it's me, its Robert. I'm home now. You're safe.' The stair cupboard door slowly opened and Ruth stepped out of the darkness, blinking slightly in the unaccustomed light. The knife was dropped to the floor and she ran to Robert's comforting arms. 'Whatever is the matter?' he said, stroking her hair gently and brushing it back from her temples. He could feel her body trembling as he led her into the kitchen and taking her hand he helped her to sit at the table. 'Come on love, tell me what's wrong. What's happened to frighten you so?'

'It's him', she replied, 'he knows where I live. Robert he knows where I live!' Ruth said becoming more and more agitated with every word. She stood up from the table and began to pace up and down. 'Did you notice anyone outside when you came in?' She asked in a hurried, breathless voice. Robert noticed that her breathing was rapid and shallow.

'Calm down, calm down, you're getting yourself into a state needlessly.' He stood up and went to her side, putting his arms around her, he pulled her to him. 'Come on, I'll make us a nice cup of tea and you can tell me what's been happening.' Robert switched the kettle on and reached for the teapot. He walked across the kitchen to collect some tea cups and as he did so he looked back at his wife. Ruth, who was now sitting back at the table, was wringing her hands furiously and still looked agitated and alarmed. Robert wondered if he ought to get her medication and then thought the better of it. Instead he chose a soothing Jack Johnson CD and put the music on quietly in the background.

They drank their tea in silence with only the sound of a gentle voice singing quietly to an acoustic guitar for company. Robert waited for Ruth's breathing to settle. She was no longer wringing her hands and looked less agitated. He felt the tension in his body ease slightly. 'The flowers are pretty,' he said. 'Would you like me to put them in water?' By accident he had stumbled onto the catalyst and Ruth began to tell him of her visits to the cemetery to put flowers on Janet's and Keith's grave.

'He's always there,' she said, 'always behind me, always watching. I've tried going in through different entrances and taking a different path through the graves. But he knows, he knows where they are and he's always waiting. And now he wants me!'

'Who wants you?' Robert asked anxiously. Ruth placed her trembling hands over her mouth and shook her head as if unwilling to speak. Robert reached out his hand and laid it on to her shoulder. 'Please darling,' he reiterated, 'who is it you're so afraid of, who wants you?'

Ruth's hands dropped from her mouth and with eyes wide with terror she blurted out, 'Death,' she said. 'Death wants me! I asked him to come for mum and now it's my turn! Oh Robert I'm so afraid.'

Chapter 10

Sean

The next morning Robert rang the doctor and made an appointment to see him. He rang Sean and asked him to come and sit with his mother while he was away. Sean duly arrived on his motorbike at the allotted time. 'How is she?' Sean asked.

'Quiet at the moment,' Robert replied. 'She's had her medication so just try and keep her calm. Talk to her about things she likes and keep her mind occupied, if you can on happy thoughts. She really is not well.'

'Don't worry Dad, I know how best to handle mum. Look I've brought this, it was going to be an anniversary present for you.' He pulled a River Dance DVD out of his pocket. "Thought I'd watch this with her,' he said. 'You know how she loves to dance.' Robert nodded and left for his appointment. Sean joined his mother in the lounge. 'How are feeling mum?' Sean asked sitting down by his mother's side on the settee and putting his arm around her shoulder. 'This cat idolises you,' he said stroking Smokey's soft grey fur. The cat was curled up, fast asleep in Ruth's lap.

Ruth turned her head to look at him and smiled warmly. Mother and son were very close. Sean, as foretold by Robert, inherited his father's looks and Ruth often used to think, it was like gazing at an old photo of a young Robert when she looked at him. The dark brown hair, the captivating blue eyes and the gentle expression behind them, were so similar. However, Sean had followed her genes in terms of stature. She was just five feet and three inches tall, while Sean was five-foot seven. He had, however, inherited his father's stocky build and made up in strength what he lacked in height.

'I brought this for us to watch,' he said, taking out the DVD. 'It's a recording of a River Dance show. I thought you might like it.'

'That was kind of you, but I'd really just like to talk,' she said resting her head on his shoulder.

'Vicky and I were wondering if you'd start teaching Francesca some ballet when you're better? Vicky's going to enrol her in the dance school in town.'

'I'd love to,' she replied, 'as soon as I get my energy reserves back. Ballet was always my favourite even from an early age. Mind you, I did love tap and ballroom dancing too. I remember when I was Francesca's age, I used to buy a girl's comic every week with my pocket money, called Bunty. One of the stories in the comic was about a ballerina who was studying at the Royal Ballet School. That was always my childhood dream, to join the Royal Ballet. I went to a dance school in Crawley three times a week until I was fourteen. I stopped going when my mum and dad's marriage started to fall apart.'

'What was the dance school called?' asked Sean trying to turn the conversation back on a positive note.

'Isabella's,' she replied, 'it was really good too.'

'Francesca makes us laugh,' Sean said. 'As soon as any music comes on the radio or the television, she starts jigging about. She looks really comical at times.'

'She's at a lovely age,' Ruth replied, 'make the most of it.'

Chapter 11

Psychic bond

'I am worried about my wife,' Robert said to the doctor, 'Since she started taking sleeping pills as well as the course of anti-depressants she is on, she's become paranoid at times. She's begun to imagine all kinds of things!'

'What kind of things?' The doctor asked.

'Well for one thing, she is convinced that...,' Robert paused for a moment and then continued, 'she thinks that death is stalking her!' He told the doctor about the events of the previous day.

When he had finished the doctor had much to say. 'It may well be that you're so in tune with your wife, that even at a distance you're able to pick up on what she is feeling and thinking, particularly in highly-charged situations. However, proof as to whether mental telepathy is a valid phenomenon is elusive. Most of the evidence is anecdotal and thus not accepted scientifically. Having said that, the anecdotal evidence is overwhelming and I have had a similar experience. My son was hurt in a car accident some years ago, but I knew instantly the moment the crash occurred that he'd been injured. So you are not alone. Mental telepathy has been well-documented if not scientifically proven.'

'We often find we are about to say the same thing at the same time. That's probably fairly common I would imagine,' said Robert interrupting, 'but when Ruth is really stressed or in some kind of crisis, I can actually see her in my mind's eye. I know what's happening to her. These last few weeks especially, since her medication has increased, I've become really fearful for her. I can sense how agitated, how distraught she is. I'm very concerned that the medication seems to be hindering her recovery more than it is helping.'

'It is becoming clearer and clearer,' the doctor went on, 'that antidepressants are far from benign drugs. Unfortunately the combination of depression and medication is still very much trial and error. Various drugs will affect patients in different ways and most patients suffer from one side affect or another. One of the most common side effects,' he continued, 'is increased anxiety and agitation. This clearly appears to be your wife's problem. What I can do is to prescribe an additional drug which ought to prevent this from happening.' Robert left the surgery with yet another prescription.

Ruth was now taking a daily cocktail of drugs which would only serve to compound her problems. Robert did not like the fact that his wife was taking so many pills, but he could only act on the advice he had been given, although it concerned him greatly. He felt that the doctor had given little guidance on how to control and in time reduce Ruth's medication and that they were being subjected to a reactive, rather than a proactive response to Ruth's problems. The weeks rolled by and Ruth showed no sign of improvement. Robert wanted to reduce her medication, but the doctor advised against it and insisted her course of treatment continue for the time being.

Chapter 12

Hallucination

A problem had arisen at work and Robert was forced to make the call he'd been trying to avoid. He phoned Ruth at about 6pm. 'I'm going to be late,' he said, 'very late.'

'How late?' she enquired.

'Could be nine o'clock or thereabouts before I'm back,' he replied.

'Just as well it's mixed salad then,' she said. 'If you don't mind I'll have mine now. The thought of taking a long, soothing lavender bath and having an early night is music to my ears. I'll plate yours up and leave it in the fridge.'

'Are you OK?' he asked, hoping for a positive response.

'Yes,' she said, 'just tired. An early night will do me good.'

'Be careful with your medication,' he said and then Ruth put the phone down.

It was shortly after 9pm when Robert pulled into the drive. He could already hear Ruth screaming, even before he was out of the car. He raced to the front door, searching frantically for the house keys in his trouser pocket. As he fumbled to fit them into the lock, they fell out of his hand. He dropped to his knees, scrabbling about in the darkness with both hands, desperately trying to find them. Ruth's screams rang shrill in the night air. Suddenly his fingers grasped metal and a shaking hand finally managed to open the front door. He raced upstairs and burst in through the bedroom door. Ruth's almost naked body was pinned against the wall above the bed and it appeared to Robert as if she was being thrust up and down by some unseen force. Her negligee had been pushed up above her breasts and her legs were splayed apart. Her hands were pressing outwards as if against the shoulders of some invisible rapist. 'Help me, for Christ's sake, help me,' she screamed. Robert shot forward to her aid and was then struck a blow, out of thin air, to his abdomen. He hurtled backwards, hitting the bedroom wall with a resounding crash. He lay on the floor, struggling for breath, whilst his wife's cries and piercing screams echoed in his ears. As he gradually managed to control his lungs once more and breathe, he watched Ruth's body, as if released from its oppressor, slide slowly down the wall and onto the bed. She curled up in a tight ball on her knees on the pillows and sobbed, crying out to him. 'Robert, Robert, please save me. Make him go away, please make him go away.' Robert struggled to his feet and went to comfort his distraught wife.

They slept, or rather did not sleep, in the guest room that night. Robert did not go into work the next day. He emptied their old bedroom of furniture and burnt what he could. He re-decorated the entire room over the next few days, but it would never again be their matrimonial bedroom. He stayed off work for two weeks and hardly left Ruth's side. He felt confused, frightened, vulnerable and degraded. He kept going over in his mind what he had seen and felt on that dreadful night. As the days wore on, he convinced himself that they must have imagined what had happened, that it couldn't possibly have taken place. He persuaded himself that blind fear had caused them both to lose sight of reality. The images in his mind of Ruth's naked body being ravaged and defiled haunted him. It was almost too awful to think about and he tried desperately to blot it out of his mind.

He telephoned Ruth's doctor to ask if the medication she was on could cause her to hallucinate. The doctor informed him that hallucination was indeed a known side effect. Robert was satisfied. This was the explanation he wanted. Ruth had been hallucinating. She had imagined herself under attack, invaded by some evil being. The strong psychic connection between them had caused Robert to experience what she had been feeling. Unwittingly he had been drawn in to, had entered her nightmare. There had been no rape. It was all in their imagination. It was the drugs, the toxic concoction of harmful chemicals which they were subjecting Ruth to each day that was to blame.

He remembered back to his University days and stories other students had told him of the darker side to LSD, of the deeply disturbing trips they experienced. Robert knew what he had to do. Somehow, Ruth had to be weaned off those drugs. Robert truly believed his theory regarding the events of that night were true. Yet, much as he tried to shut them out, images of it still haunted him. He told no-one, not even Sean about their experience and even he and Ruth avoided all conversation about that terrible night. They skirted around the subject, as if they were novice climbers traversing around a crevasse on a mountain glacier.

Chapter 13

The overdose

Robert reluctantly returned to work. Then one evening in late-January he arrived home to find the house in darkness. It was unusual for Ruth not be in when he arrived back from work. Even though she had been unwell she had always been waiting for him and he could tell she was pleased to have him home again. She would often say she didn't like being alone, that was when she had her darkest thoughts. Robert parked the car and walked up to the front door. Taking out his key he turned it in the lock and opening the door reached inside for the light switch in the hall. He pressed the switch several times but the light did not come on. It was so pitch black that he had to feel his way along the hall to locate the lounge door. He pushed it open. Once again his fingers searched for the light switch and finding it, he pressed again. Then it came to him they must have had a power cut. Feeling his way past the furniture in the lounge he went into the kitchen and groped for the cupboard door on the far wall, inside which was their electricity meter. On opening the cupboard door and looking at the meter he was surprised to see that the trip switch had not blown and the meter light was still flashing. Clearly the house had full power. He continued to try all the lights in every one of the downstairs rooms but not one light was working. 'I need a torch' he thought to himself, and went out to the garage to collect one.

When he returned, he shone the torch at the light fitting in the kitchen. There was no bulb. He was soon to discover that in every room in the house the light bulb had been removed. The bathroom upstairs was the last

The Grim Reaper

room he checked. The door was locked. Ruth was inside in total darkness. He could not get her to talk or to open the door and spent an uncomfortable night on the landing. As daylight returned, finally he heard the bathroom lock turn and Ruth emerged through the door onto the landing. She was dressed all in black. He heard himself asking if she was OK. She nodded. 'I'm alright now,' she said, 'I just wanted to be invisible.' All the light bulbs were in the bath. Robert returned them to their respective fittings and rang Sean. 'I have to go to work today Sean but I don't like leaving your mother. She's not well.'

'Sorry Dad,' replied Sean,' but Vicky's away at her mum's and I've got the kids all day.'

'Never mind,' replied Robert,' I'll just have to get back early today.'

When he returned home from work he found Ruth unconscious on the kitchen floor, her bottle of sleeping pills lay empty on the table beside her. Ruth had been taking anti-depressant pills for months, which had caused her to suffer from insomnia and anxiety. To counteract this unwanted side-effect, she had been prescribed sleeping tablets by the doctor. She was taking this combination of drugs for months. The problem was that the longer she had been taking the tablets, the more she needed for them to take effect.

Robert immediately rang for an ambulance. He then poured water into a large glass and emptied a good measure of salt into it. He pulled Ruth up into a sitting position and began forcibly to make her drink. Within minutes she was choking and vomiting. When the ambulance arrived, she was taken to hospital, where she was stomach pumped. On returning to the accident and emergency ward she was given a private room and

Robert sat by her bedside all night. The next morning, Robert managed to convince the doctors that Ruth's overdose had been a mistake and several days later she was allowed home. Robert never forgave himself for the fact that she had taken an overdose of sleeping pills and could so easily have died. He sometimes had nightmares reliving that night, only this time arriving home even later and finding Ruth dead. It was then that he made his decision to retire early. Robert was never quite sure whether the overdose had been intentional or not. He hoped rather than believed that it was accidental.

Chapter 14

Ruth's recovery

However, little by little, with his loving care Ruth began to get well. Her medication was reduced and Robert began to feel more and more optimistic about the future. Ruth was laughing again and her appetite was back. She no longer looked so gaunt and thin. For the first time over recent weeks Robert noticed how happy she was in the company of her grandchildren. Sean married two years before Keith died and was now the proud father of a three year-old girl called Francesca and a ten-month old baby girl called Freya. His wife Victoria was fond of Ruth and helped Robert enormously, staying with Ruth if he had to go away or if Sean wanted to spend the day out biking with his dad. The love of motorbikes and cycling had been passed from father to son.

Recently Vicky volunteered to stay with Ruth for two whole weeks. Francesca was delighted at the prospect of staying with Granny and Smokey for an extended stay. Sean finally managed to persuade his father to complete the famous John O'Groat's to Land's End cycle ride. Sean had been desperate to do this ride since he was a teenager and now at last, with Ruth much recovered; father and son had decided the time was right. It had taken fifteen days to complete the ride, cycling in total over 1600 kilometres and with an average of 108 kilometres per day. Robert telephoned Ruth every evening and listened with warm satisfaction how Ruth had spent her day with her two granddaughters. In the two weeks he and Sean were away, she had even been swimming on four separate occasions with Vicky and the girls and, on her own, had taken Francesca to her dance classes. This was progress indeed. As for Robert and Sean they were in their element cycling together and having a fantastic time. The physical exercise did them the power of good and they returned home looking toned and fit. On their return Robert noticed how bright-eyed and bushy-tailed his wife looked. 'Could life really be returning to normal?' he asked himself and for the first time in a long time, he felt hope. It was a joyous reunion.

Ruth, who was an excellent cook, excelled herself. She cooked Robert's favourite meal consisting of a homemade mushroom soup, roast lamb with all the trimmings and a Swiss apple tart. If there was one thing for which Ruth had a well-deserved reputation in the kitchen it was her pastry making. Her pastry was always crisp, rich and delicious. She tried to teach Vicky and in fairness Vicky's pastry had improved. However, it was Ruth who remained the unrivalled master of both the short crust and puff varieties. For the first few nights Ruth and Vicky delighted in listening to tales of their respective husbands' many exploits during their trip. They also raised £800 for cancer relief in memory of Janet, and Ruth told Robert several times how proud she was of him.

To Robert, Ruth was still beautiful, but the ravages of the heartache she experienced in the manner of her father's passing and the subsequent ill-health she had suffered since his death, had taken its toll. The once thick head of black hair had vanished and in its place, lank thinning strands of grey, punctuated here and there with rogue streaks of white, now framed the loved and familiar face. When Robert had first introduced Ruth to his mother and sister, it was her diminutive size and the striking green eyes which they had noticed first. Ruth's eyes had been uniquely beautiful and to the envy of his sister, they were bordered by the thickest, darkest lashes she had ever seen. Who needed mascara with lashes like that? But it was the expression behind the eyes that fascinated most, an unequivocal look of kindness and compassion, of wanting to accept and be accepted. Both mother and sister had determined on disliking Robert's choice of a first love, but they had been captivated by her within minutes of meeting.

'What did you think of her?' Robert asked later.

'She's a treasure,' Peggy answered, 'very pretty and a lovely figure.'

'Well, she'll certainly be easy to carry over the threshold, that's for certain,' his sister had added in conclusion.

Chapter 15

Elizabeth

Throughout their early years brother and sister had been devoted to one another. They sought sanctuary in each other's company from the theatre of war which seemed to envelop their family life. Robert's sister, Elizabeth, was three years his junior and for the first five years of her life, he and Peggy were the centre of her universe. Elizabeth idolised her big brother and would do anything he asked. He had persuaded her that large copper coins were more valuable than the smaller silver ones she received in her pocket money. It made sense to her, that size denoted value. She would happily exchange her silver coins for bronze, with the brother she looked up to almost as a father figure. Elizabeth worshipped the very ground Robert walked on. She grew up believing that he had all the qualities she lacked and she desperately tried to follow his example. He was determined, never gave up on anything and would stick with any and every project, until he made it right. She, in contrast, would flit from one interest to another and as soon as a problem arose she would move on and leave the problem behind and unattended to. He was as resolute as she was unreliable and she envied his controlled manner and logical mind. She was often illogical and wild in her behaviour.

Elizabeth was fully aware of the division between her father and her brother. She was always saddened by the conflict and often tried to act as an intermediary, explaining the actions of one to the other and trying to find common ground to resolve their differences. Elizabeth always felt that father and son had much more in common with one another than they realised. Her

The Grim Reaper

father had been starved of affection as a child growing up in a family of thirteen and with his mother going from one pregnancy straight into another. They had been as poor as church mice, often going without food and without any form of heating in the long cold winters her father had described to her. Robert too had been deprived a mother's affection because of George's inability to share his wife with his own children. It had been a vicious circle, what had gone around had come around again. Elizabeth could see the sadness of their situation but felt helpless to resolve or repair it. As Robert grew to manhood she was saddened still further, by George's decline in status in the household. He was no longer the alpha male, Robert had taken on that role and George's already low self-esteem and unhappiness was even more prevalent.

She wished with all her heart that Robert could learn to love his father and forgive the sins of the past. Elizabeth knew that Robert was capable of exceptional love, after all she had his love and she had seen the devotion he also felt, for his favourite Aunt and Uncle. It was a devotion that was all too obvious at times. Whenever they visited, he would behave as if they were his real parents and she often caught sight of the terrible sadness and regret that both George and Peggy displayed at such times. Robert was particularly close to his Uncle Jack. Uncle Jack had a motorbike with a side-car and even before he was three years old Robert was a seasoned passenger.

Elizabeth believed that Robert had decided to own a bike himself, before he had even been weaned and that he had started saving up to buy it, even before he could walk. Whilst they had been at junior school together, every Wednesday Robert would take Elizabeth to a fish and chip shop for lunch. The shop was situated just yards outside the school gate. Every other day they went home on the bus for lunch. But, on Wednesday's Peggy would visit her older sister, who lived out in the country. Robert was given money to buy their chip shop dinner. For three years, Elizabeth had a bag of scratchins for lunch, which cost Robert a single penny. They would sit together on a bench overlooking the Stour River munching the crispy batter and Elizabeth thought she was in heaven.

From the age of six, Robert held down two paper rounds and worked weekends at a local pub, bottling up. The day after his 17th birthday he bought his first motor bike, with his by now ample savings. From that day on Robert and his bike were inseparable. The bike proved to be another cause of arguments between Robert and his father. George objected to the bike residing in the living room. Robert would often wheel his beloved motorbike into the house and spend days dismantling and rebuilding it in the middle of the family living room. George was not impressed.

Elizabeth remembered the day of Robert's first motorcycle test. He bought her a helmet and promised to take her for a ride as soon as he returned home. She waited all day. Robert left early in the morning to go to the test centre. He passed everything and all that remained was his demonstration of an emergency stop. Mr Deakin, the examiner, asked him to do a continuous circle of the roads around Crawley Abbey. At some point, he explained, he would ask Robert to demonstrate his emergency stop. Three quarters of an hour later, Robert called back at the test centre to inform them he was running low on petrol. He needed to let Mr Deakin know that he would be back in five minutes. The gentleman he spoke to on the reception desk informed him that Mr Deakin had been run over by a motorbike and had gone off to hospital in an ambulance some time ago.

Elizabeth did get her first ride, but not that day. Over the years she was a regular passenger and she loved being out on the bike with him. In her eyes, Robert more than made up for his early unethical, entrepreneurial skills. He taught her to play chess and football, climb trees, ride a bike and become an expert on roller skates. Most importantly he taught her to appreciate her own talents. He made her brave, fearless and she met every physical challenge head on. He also made her a tomboy. She liked cars and trains, bows and arrows, cowboy hats, cap guns and pea-shooters. Dolls and dolls' prams remained unused in the toy cupboard. As they grew older the differences in abilities between them became more pronounced. She showed herself to be gifted in art and modern languages, whereas he was gifted, like his mother, in the Sciences and Mathematics. The speed at which mother and son could add up a column of figures was to Elizabeth incredible.

She also remembered that Christmases throughout their childhood were the highlight of the year. Peggy was one of five siblings and whilst they never mixed with George's side of the family, every Christmas Peggy's family would gather together, in either their home or in the home of Peggy's eldest sister. These were magical times and brother and sister felt part of a strong and vibrant family. Robert in particular determined that he would establish his own loving family and that it would be equally as strong, if not more so than his mother's. Robert was particularly close to Peggy's youngest sister and her husband. His Aunt Mary and Uncle Jack, both of whom were devout Christians, lost their only son. He had been still born. For them, Robert became almost a replacement child and he was devoted to them both. His

Uncle's love of motorbikes and of travelling planted a seed in Robert's childhood. That seed would flourish and a love of motorbikes and travel would stay with him throughout his life.

Chapter 16

Love at first sight

Ruth was definitely on the mend, hence Robert's reason for organising the holiday. She was almost off medication altogether and Robert hoped that a day out in the fresh air doing what they loved best, would see her get a good night's sleep, without the need of sleeping tablets. He felt the day was proving to be a success and was congratulating himself on his decision to take Ruth on a short break. His only regret on the day so far was that they were not on the bike. When Ruth and Robert had met, she quickly discovered his passion for motorbikes. He reminded her of a fanatical rocker, clad as he was in his black leather biker's outfit. Ruth had been more of a mod and had been planning on buying a scooter. She owned several pairs of white knee length boots and often wore flowers in her long black hair. She certainly had a flower power mentality and was against the atom bomb and all wars. The old saying that opposites attract might well be true, but in terms of attitude if not dress, they were absolutely identical. They had the same likes and dislikes, the same interests and needs. In truth, they were kindred spirits. Within days of their meeting, Ruth's mod clothes had vanished. Instead, two young people dressed in their leathers would head off on the open highway every weekend. Ruth would be glued to Robert's back. They and the bike had become one and more importantly they had fixed each other. Everything that had been missing in their lives, they now had in abundance.

They had met at the Crawley Flower Show in 1965. This annual event is held in mid- August over two days (in recent times Friday and Saturday) at the Riverside, the main park in Crawley situated right on the banks of the River Stour. The show is one of the largest events of its type in the United Kingdom and is also one of the longest running shows in the world. Visitors from home and abroad flock to see the wonderful displays on offer and to admire the natural scenery. It is hardly surprising therefore that the show is often described as an event in which 'Nature competes with contrived beauty.' The park is really magnificent and is set in long, green, sweeping fields which stretch down to the reeds and bulrushes of the banks of the majestic River Stour.

The park has a formal sunken garden called The Dell, containing colourful herbaceous borders punctuated with sculptured green lawns and decorated with sparkling fountains and marble statues. There are rock pools built into its steep sides, containing myriads of gold fish. Each rock pool is equipped with stepping stones or a little wooden bridge to cross and the pools themselves are linked together with rough cut stone paths for the intrepid explorer to investigate. At the centre of the Dell is a large landscaped lake. The lake itself is home to a wide variety of ducks, swans and geese enjoying its clear but lily patched waters. The show is set out under a large number of marquees over the 29-acre land area of the Riverside. Inside the marquees are displays of flowers, fruit, vegetables and a fine array of arts and crafts work. An outdoor arena hosts a number of spectacular events from show jumping, motor cycle display teams, gymnastic displays and military marching bands. A Victorian bandstand with views over the river is used to stage a variety of musical and variety acts and the show culminates in a fantastic evening firework display. The firework display is an event not to be missed and causes great excitement in the town every year.

The Grim Reaper

On this particular Saturday, Robert had been at the Show with a number of school friends. They had been standing in the main spectator area, outside the central arena watching an act called 'The Ariel Karindas.' This was a high wire act, 100 feet up with no safety net and consisted of a uni-cyclist performing various balancing acts. Every head but one was looking up. Robert had spotted Ruth in the crowd, standing with some girl friends just yards to his left. He could not take his eyes off her and even if the Ariel Karindas had fallen off the wire, Robert's eyes would have remained firmly fixed on Ruth. The act finished and the vast crowds started to disperse and move away. One of Robert's friends caught his arm and pointed to the beer tent. 'Pasty and a pint, what do you reckon?' he asked. By the time Robert had declined and looked round to see where Ruth was, she had vanished. The rest of the day seemed to drag to Robert. Everywhere he and his friends went, nothing was of interest. He wanted to see Ruth's face in the crowd, to introduce himself and to speak to her. He simply had to know her name.

He excused himself from his friends and systematically searched every marquee, but to no avail. He walked the river bank for the entire length of the park. Many pretty girls decorated the lush green grass lining the water's edge, but the girl with long black hair, dressed in a red PVC mackintosh and wearing white knee length boots was nowhere to be seen. Robert reluctantly rejoined his friends and half-heartedly watched the events taking place in the main arena. However, the Show Jumping and even the motor cycle display team had little interest for him. They moved to the bandstand to watch the variety acts, but he barely noticed the jugglers act, or the plate spinner. Instead his eyes constantly searched the crowd for sight of her. He hardly heard the comments of his friends and his ears were deaf too, to the songs of the many male voice choirs and to the music of musical bands which filled the air with a cacophony of sound. Thrice more he parted company with his friends and walked through the Dell, hoping to find her admiring the flower borders or watching the ducks on the lake but, it was as if she had vanished into thin air.

Night had fallen and Robert had almost given up hope of ever seeing her again. He and his friends were back where they had been earlier in the day, in the main spectator area outside the central arena in which the firework display was due to start. As the first giant sky rocket exploded in a blaze of light, he saw her. Ruth's face was suddenly lit up in a golden glow. Robert left his friends and made his way towards her, until standing right by her side. 'Do you like fireworks?' he said.

She turned to look at him and smiled. 'Love them,' she replied.

'What about the Beatles?' he asked.

'Do you mean of the Liverpudlian variety?' she asked eagerly.

'What other variety is there?' he said with a broad smile.

'Love them too,' she replied with an even wider smile, which melted his heart in seconds. 'Why do you ask?'

'Thought you might like to come and see the film Help with me tomorrow? My name's Robert, Robert Weston by the way. What's yours?'

'Ruth, Ruth Evans' she answered, blushing slightly, 'and yes I'd love to see Help with you.'

The Grim Reaper

'Ruth,' he repeated, 'do you realise we might have the same initials one day!'

'Gosh you're not backward in coming forward are you,' she said jokingly.

'Not when I see something I want,' he answered, looking her straight in the eyes. The firework display continued. The night sky was lit up time and time again with loud, colourful explosions. Sparks of red, green, purple and gold rained down upon them and Robert watched their reflection in the sleek, shining blackness of her hair.

'Would you like to walk me home?' she said when they finally realised that all their friends had left without them.

'I'd like to walk you home every night from now on,' he replied, taking her hand in his.

'I think that could be arranged,' Ruth said smiling up at a young man she had only just met. She ought to have felt she was with a complete stranger, but she didn't. She felt she had known this young man forever and Robert too was feeling as if his ship had reached safe harbour. It was love at first sight for both of them and nothing on earth, nothing they would ever face in life would have the power to separate them. It would be a relationship that would live up to the title of Ruth's favourite film and could certainly be penned - a love affair to remember.

Chapter 17

Rug Chapel

Ruth and Robert walked slowly back to the car enjoying the warm sunshine and taking one last look at beautiful Bala, they resumed their journey. They decided to visit Rug Chapel situated in glorious countryside at the foot of the Berwyn Mountain's and just west of the historic town of Corwen. Robert booked bed and breakfast accommodation overnight at an old coaching Inn in the centre of Corwen. The Inn was in easy walking distance of several sites of historic interest, including the motte of a Norman Castle and the famous bronze statue of Owain Glyndwr, the 15th century Welsh prince who led the Welsh in their struggle for independence. They were listening to an old Led Zeppelin CD as they arrived at the church singing the lyrics to 'Stairway to Heaven.' 'Oh don't switch it off.' Ruth requested. 'I love this song.' The song finished and Robert turned off the engine. Looking at the chapel he felt strangely disappointed. He opened the passenger door and helped Ruth out into the warm sunshine. 'What lovely views!' she exclaimed looking around.

Robert was also pleased with the location, but the chapel to him looked very small and plain. Rug chapel had been built in 1637 as a private worship house for the Salisbury family. It was surrounded by rolling green hills. Grazing sheep dotted the landscape and rose hedges divided a tapestry of arable fields and water meadows. The meadows were seemingly devoid of life, except for an array of noisy wild birds, soaring high above the lush grasses. A blackthorn hedgerow, ablaze with white flowers lined perimeter of the churchyard as well as one side of a steep rocky path which lead down

The Grim Reaper

to the chapel door. Avoiding the hedges razor sharp thorns they made their down to the large oak doors. From the outside the small slate chapel had appeared quite plain, but inside there was much craftsmanship to be admired.

Although only a small out-of-the way chapel, Robert was not disappointed once inside. Every surface had been decorated with paintings, carvings or both. Robert's eyes found themselves drawn to the ceiling and he gasped. The impressive ceiling was incredibly ornate. Every truss and panel had been painted with swirls of blue or red vine roses. The famous Rug angels, wooden cut-outs painted in blues, greens, reds and gold seemed to hover above Robert's head. The angels were fixed to the roof trusses and appeared as if they were flying. A wooden chandelier in the shape of another angel with a wide skirt of candle holders was also suspended from the high ceiling. Robert thought to himself that he would have liked to have seen it with its candles lit.

A rood screen richly engraved with angels that would have separated the clergy from the congregation was the next thing to catch his eye. Ruth also noticed the elaborate roof. She pointed out the ends of the beams which were decorated with intertwining rose motifs. Everywhere they looked they could see superb carvings from the altar rail, the family pews, painted gallery and even to the bench ends. The long 'running' boards that connected the bottoms of the pews were particularly fascinating. Robert noted that each one had been carved with a mythological or Christian beast. He could see carvings of pelicans, griffins, dragons and serpents. Ruth seemed fascinated in a ghoulish wall painting of a recumbent skeleton. The death painting featured a skeleton, hourglass, a sundial and burning candles, all symbols of the transience of life and the coming of death. 'Oh,' said Robert studying it closely, 'makes me shiver, I don't like the look of him at all.'

'Yes,' said Ruth 'but I think it serves the artist's purpose in reminding us of our mortality and as a warning.'

'Why do you say warning?' Robert inquired.

'Well yes, a warning,' Ruth replied, 'in that we better be good while we are on Earth if we want our reward in heaven, when death finally takes us.'

Chapter 18

The figure of death

At that moment an old lady who had entered the church shortly after their arrival asked if they were interested in seeing another small chapel. It was only a short walk away and much older than Rug by the name of Llangar. 'It's a medieval building with lovely views overlooking the confluence of the Dee and Alwen rivers, and if you've got time on your hands it would be a worthwhile visit,' she continued. They followed behind her at a short distance as she led them down a narrow track towards a coppice at the back of Rug Chapel and then on across lush meadows leading down into a green valley of patchwork fields. The setting was truly idyllic. In the distance, Robert could see where the two rivers joined and admired a unique view. Wide, fast-flowing waters sparkled with dazzling brilliance in the bright afternoon sunshine. In the background, green fields set against a backdrop of rugged mountains created a colourful and interesting landscape. The whitewashed church, however, appeared very isolated. Robert noted immediately how steep the path was leading down to its ancient wooden doors. He instinctively took hold of Ruth's hand. They descended through the steeply sloping churchyard passing between jumbled tiers of tombstones. The stones were encrusted with lichen. There were no flowers on any of the graves and Robert felt as if the little church had been abandoned and forgotten and left to decay.

Robert was also by this time feeling a little annoyed with the old lady. Ruth was only just recovering from her illness and was not used to so much exercise. The last thing he wanted was for her to be overly tired. As with

Rug, this chapel seemed to have little to offer from the outside. They stood outside the large oak doors whilst the old lady reached into her coat pocket to find a very old brass key with a strangely wrought handle. The shape of the handle resembled two concentric circles joined in the centre by a serpent. The door creaked as the old lady pushed it open and as Robert ushered Ruth in ahead of him he noticed an unusual rough carving on the doors themselves. They too had been engraved with the symbol of two concentric circles with an odd looking motif etched into the eye at the centre. 'According to legend,' the old lady said, 'the church was originally named 'Llan Garw Gwyn,' the church of the white stag, after the appearance of a magical deer. The locals were so awed they established a church on the same spot.'

The chapel felt cold and damp inside and had none of the interior riches waiting to greet the visitor at Rug. Plain beams, box pews and pulpit afforded little opportunity to admire an artist's hand, although there were extensive if somewhat fading 15th century wall paintings as well as a 17th century figure of death. There was a towering three-decker pulpit and Robert wondered whether the sermons would have been enlightening – or whether they had tended more towards the fire and brimstone variety. He suspected the latter. It was a very large pulpit best suited to a larger than life personality. He noted the box pews where the gentry would have been seated and the rough benches for lesser mortals. At one end of the church was the altar covered with Georgian style furnishings and at the other a minstrel's gallery, with a four-sided music stand. The church had a medieval timber roof with a barrel-vaulted 'canopy of honour' over the altar. The wall paintings were of medieval saints and depictions of deadly sins. He recognised gluttony, fornication, lust, greed and despair and the painting of wrath was frightening to behold. Like Rug chapel, this church also had a wall painting of the Grim Reaper. The skeleton was standing upright, holding a spear and an hourglass. Depicted behind him were the tools of a gravedigger, the pickaxe and the spade. Robert felt his body shudder in the chill atmosphere.

Robert was looking at this image of the Grim Reaper when he noticed Ruth climbing up some steps which led to the minstrel's gallery. Instantly, he felt something was wrong. The hairs on the back of his neck stood up and another sudden chill ran through his body. He turned quickly and called out to Ruth. 'Come down darling, we ought to be moving on, it's later than I thought.' Ruth did not reply. He called to her again, noting that she had turned to face the wall and as he looked up at her it seemed to him that dark shapes were moving in the air around her. As he watched almost rooted to the spot for a moment he noticed her hair was rising and lifting off her shoulders although the air in the chapel was completely still. He raced up the steps and ran to grab her. The dark shapes he had seen swirling about her seemed to vanish in an instant. Ruth was staring at an oak wall covered in rough carvings of the same concentric circles he had noticed on the door. Taking her hand with his now trembling hand he gently pulled her down the steps, anxious to be away. The old lady was waiting just inside the door and Robert observed the oddest of expressions on her face. When he tried to describe it to Sean later he could only say it was one of pure evil combined with absolute satisfaction.

Robert led the way back to the car holding tightly on to Ruth's hand, the old lady following at a safe distance behind. As they neared Rug Chapel where the car was parked Robert glanced back and noticed that the old woman was now nowhere in sight. He opened the passenger door to the car and helped Ruth inside. Robert felt incredibly anxious. He tried to engage Ruth in conversation as they had walked back along the path but she was silent throughout. She looked pale and drawn and the dark circles around her eyes which had been fading, now once again contrasted starkly with the sickly pallor of her skin. 'It's home for us,' Robert thought to himself.

Chapter 19

Ruth's isolation

For the whole of the drive Ruth remained silent. She looked neither right nor left, simply staring straight ahead but as if not seeing, almost as if she was in a trance like state. Robert telephoned Sean as soon as they were back. They cooked tea together discussing the events of the day in low voices. Ruth sat in the lounge. Her eyes appeared focused on the cat flap at the bottom of the front door. Neither Robert nor Sean could get her to talk, she was completely unresponsive. They brought her a tray with some food on it and placed it on her lap. Even Robert found he had difficulty in swallowing, his stomach felt in knots, but Ruth ate nothing at all. It must have been about 9 o'clock when Robert stooped to take the untouched tray from Ruth's lap. Just as he did so, Smokey, their Persian cat entered at her usual leisurely pace through the cat flap. The cat, immediately recognising its mistress, ran across the carpet towards Ruth's chair. Suddenly and without warning it stopped dead in its tracks, claws stuck into the carpet as it arched its back, gave an alarming hiss and then ripping its claws free it shot back out through the cat flap.

Sean stayed later that night than he had intended. He urged his father to call the doctor, but Robert insisted on letting Ruth get a good night's sleep. 'I'll see how she is in the morning and if there's no improvement, I'll ring the surgery straight away,' he promised. Robert never knew exactly what the time was that night when he woke up in a cold sweat. His explanation to Sean was that he must have been having a nightmare. He had woken up suddenly with a jolt to find his pyjamas were soaked in perspiration. He immediately looked over in the darkness at his wife lying beside him and saw the figure of the Grim Reaper standing right next to the bed, leaning over her.

The tall cloaked figure seemed to be staring at Ruth. Its head, which was tilted down slightly was covered by a dark hood, the face and eyes completely hidden from Robert's view. The Reaper stood unmoving and then as if sensing Robert was watching him, the head began to lift up. Slowly, very slowly the awful pallid, sallow face was revealed. Robert would never forget its ghastly colour or the hollow eyes. The eyes were black, jet black, sunken and with heavy drooping lids. But it was the expression in the eyes which froze Robert to his very core. It was an expression of an evil, malicious intent and a look of absolute contempt. So disturbing was the visage that Robert wanted to look away, but found himself unable to do so. Whilst the eyes stared down upon him he found it impossible to turn away. The Reaper slowly raised his arms and as he did he seemed to glide silently back from Ruth's bedside. Robert watched the figure fade away as if it had evaporated through the bedroom wall. He sat upright in bed and reached out to switch on the bedside light. His heart was racing and he had difficulty breathing. He felt as if his chest had been compressed with an iron band and his whole body was trembling.

The light remained on all night. Robert did not sleep. Ruth, however, slept all night and much to Robert's relief she seemed a little better when morning finally arrived. She did not touch her cereal at breakfast, but her cup of tea was drunk to the last dregs. Throughout the day, Robert kept going back over in his mind what had happened in the chapel. He convinced himself he must have been having a bad dream, that somehow the

The Grim Reaper

image of the figure of death he had seen on the walls at Llangar played tricks on his mind, making him imagine that it had been standing over Ruth in the night. He did not call the doctor.

That afternoon Sean arrived with his family. Robert once more had reason to be concerned when Ruth directly left the room and going upstairs asked to be left alone to rest. She did not even acknowledge her grandchildren. Francesca was particularly upset and had wanted to show her grandmother some new dance steps she had learnt. 'Can you tell granny I've learnt some new steps granddad?' Francesca asked several times during the afternoon. Robert tried to oblige her but Ruth was unresponsive. When the family left Robert tried to persuade Ruth to come down into the kitchen and have something to eat. 'I'm not hungry,' she replied, 'I seem to have lost my appetite.'

'Well, you must have something,' Robert insisted, 'you've had nothing since lunch yesterday.' He took another tray of food up to Ruth and sat quietly with her watching her move the food around the plate with her fork. She ate a very little.

'Sorry,' she said, 'I really can't eat any more. You go down and watch television for a while. I'm going to have an early night.' Robert needed no persuasion. He stayed up past midnight and when he eventually entered the bedroom as quietly as he could for fear of waking her, he found Ruth sitting upright in bed, wide awake and staring at a full moon which seemed to be right up against their window. He drew the curtains closed, coaxed her into lying down and suggested sleep would be a good thing for both of them. He went to kiss her goodnight but she turned her head away and he found himself gently kissing the side of her forehead.

'Everything will be alright,' he said reassuringly, 'get some sleep.' Robert awoke three times in the night and every time Ruth was sitting up in bed staring out at the moon and with the bedroom curtains drawn back again. It was a disturbed night for them both.

Chapter 20

Voices

Robert woke up late, it had gone 9.30am. Ruth was now fast asleep. He got out of bed as carefully as he could so as not to wake her. He was convinced she would get better if only he could get her to rest and eat. He went downstairs, breakfasted and then started to prepare her favourite casserole. At 1pm Robert went back upstairs to check on his wife. Ruth was standing naked in front of the bedroom mirror with a pair of nail scissors in her right hand. As she turned to face him Robert was horrified to see that she had scratched two concentric circles on her abdomen. 'Ruth, my God what have you done to yourself?' he said in a startled voice and snatching the scissors out of her hand he ran to the medicine cabinet in the bathroom. He returned quickly and dressed the wound as best he could and then helped her into some loose clothes from her wardrobe. A long silence later, Robert finding it impossible to express his worry and concern, the casserole he had lovingly prepared was served but unappreciated. Ruth hardly touched a mouthful. She sat quietly all afternoon in the lounge, hardly speaking. She was distant, subdued and yet strangely calm. There was still no sign of Smokey's return and Robert was amazed that Ruth had not mentioned her. Smokey was Ruth's cat and she adored her. Robert suggested they go out for a walk to get some fresh air. 'Some exercise might bring your appetite back and we can look for Smokey while we're out.'

'You go,' she replied, 'I think I might read a book.' Robert walked the neighbourhood for about an hour and called on several neighbours who had looked after the cat whilst Ruth and he had been away for any length of time. No one had seen the cat. Robert returned home disappointed that he did not have any good news for Ruth. He entered through the gate leading to the back door at the rear of the house and was surprised to find Ruth outside in the garden. To his alarm he noticed straightaway that she had a large pair of garden secateurs in her hand. 'I've finished now,' she said, walking past him and placing the secateurs in his hand before stepping back through the kitchen door into the house. Robert watched her go and then surveyed the garden with dismay. He had planted an array of spring bulbs when they first moved into the house all those years ago. Over the years they had spread and the garden in the height of spring was a blaze of colour. The herbaceous borders were normally packed with row upon row of tulips and daffodils of many different varieties providing a glorious display of red, pink and yellow blooms. Not one flower head had been left. All had been cut off and lay trodden into the soil. Only green leaves and decapitated stems remained.

Robert went back into the house. He found Ruth sitting on a chair in the lounge staring into space. He knelt down on the floor by her side and gently placed his hand on her knee. 'What did you do that for, love?' he asked. 'What made you cut all the flower heads off?'

'The voices,' she replied, 'the voices told me to!'

'What voices?' Robert asked even more anxiously.

'They're in my head all the time, all the time, they don't stop, whispering, whispering and whispering.'

'What are they whispering?' Robert continued.

The Grim Reaper

'Bad things, always bad things' and with that she brought her finger to her lips and whispered so quietly that Robert could only just make out what she said. 'They want me to be quiet now,' and with that she became silent and withdrawn again.

Later that evening Robert had an idea he hoped might draw Ruth out of herself. Sean had bought them a River Dance DVD as an anniversary present which as yet they had not watched. Some while ago they both viewed a documentary on how River Dance had come about and Ruth, who loved to dance herself, loved this particularly unique style. Robert promised to take her to a live show one day. He switched the television on, inserted the disc into the DVD player and pressed 'play'. He expected to immediately hear lively, energetic Irish music, but instead a weird and plaintive sound emanated from the television and an eerie, haunting melody filled the room.

As he looked at the television screen he watched the show begin. The stage curtains were slowly drawn back to reveal a single dancer dressed in a Grim Reaper costume. For a few seconds he watched the dancer move across the stage with a series of odd jerky movements. The camera then seemed to zoom in on the dancer's face. Dark sunken eyes seemed to bulge out of the screen and black lips set in a sickly white complexion opened widely to mime a silent scream. The camera drew back and Robert watched the Grim Reaper make a slow full turn and then point out at the audience with the finger of a long bony hand. As he pointed out to the 4th wall in the centre of the stage, Robert had the most disconcerting feeling. He felt convinced that the dancer was pointing and looking at him. The DVD was switched off and Robert turned to look at Ruth. She was on her feet, her mouth wide-opened and the index finger of her right hand was pointing straight at him.

Chapter 21

Smokey's fate

Robert rang Sean from the kitchen and asked him to call round. He put the phone down and began to prepare supper with hands that were unusually shaky. Ruth joined Robert in the kitchen. He managed to raise a weak smile and put on a Wings tape for them to listen to, trying to establish some sort of normality. The doorbell rang and Robert went to let Sean in. 'When your mum has gone to bed I need to talk to you,' Robert said sounding worried and anxious. 'Try and help me get her to eat something,' he concluded just as the music stopped. They returned to the kitchen to find Ruth standing in front of the granite worktop with a kitchen knife held up high in her right hand. Her left hand was laid flat on top of the work-surface. Before Robert or Sean could do anything Ruth brought the knife down sharply. She made no sound, she did not scream, they could hear the metal cutting through bone and sinew and the final chink as the blade struck granite. Both rushed to her aid. 'Don't try removing the knife, get me a towel and ring for an ambulance,' Robert yelled horrified by what he had just witnessed. 'This is my fault. I should have done something sooner.' Robert went in the ambulance with Ruth to hospital and Sean followed behind in his car. It seemed a never-ending journey as Robert tried to keep the towel and the padding the ambulance crew had given him around the knife. He and Ruth were covered in blood.

'You did the right thing to leave the knife in,' said the staff nurse as she and two other nurses wheeled Ruth away on a trolley to a treatment room. As Ruth disappeared out of view Robert collapsed on to the floor at Sean's feet. 'Come on Dad,' Sean said lifting his father up, 'let's get you a hot cup of tea.'

'I think I need something stronger than that,' Robert replied visibly shaking. They were sitting sipping their tea in a waiting room and Robert was speaking to Sean in a hushed whisper. 'Something happened in that church. There was this rune, a sign carved into the wood everywhere you looked. It made me feel uneasy and I could see shapes moving around her when she went up to that gallery. Sean, I feel like I'm losing her and I'm frightened for her. The way she's behaving it's just not normal. I've never known her like this before even when she was ill. It's almost as if she's been possessed by an evil spirit intent on causing harm and everywhere I look I seem to see the Grim Reaper.'

Sean listened in silence for a moment and then said, 'Surely you don't believe in all that demonic possession stuff do you?'

'I don't know what I believe any more,' Robert said putting his head in his hands. 'Oh God, please help me.'

Ruth was to be kept in overnight and Robert was to ring the next morning to see what time he could speak with the doctor. 'Can I speak with her before we go home?' he asked.

'She's sedated,' the nurse replied, 'we thought it best.'

'Do you want me to stay with you?' Sean asked as he dropped his father off at home.

'No I'll be fine,' Robert replied 'and anyway it wouldn't be fair on Vicky and the kids. I'll call you tomorrow.' Robert turned the key in the lock and went inside. He switched the lights on and immediately went into the kitchen. He began to mop up the blood on the worktop

The Grim Reaper

and on the floor and when everything was pristine clean, he finally washed his hands clean of Ruth's blood. Picking up an empty cardboard box from the cupboard under the stairs, he went back to the kitchen and removed every kitchen knife he could find. He checked every draw. Finally, Robert took a reel of sellotape from the desk in his office and wrapped layer after layer around the box. Once he was satisfied it was secure, he made his way out to the garage. He pushed open the door, switched on the light and carried the box across to a wall cabinet on one side of the garage where he stored his DIY tools. The box containing knives was put on the bottom shelf and pushed right to the back. He breathed a sigh of relief and turned around. The sigh was followed by a loud gasp as his eyes caught sight of Smokey. The now dead cat was nailed by its front paws to the back of the garage door.

Robert went back into the kitchen and poured himself a stiff drink. Two more drinks later the whisky bottle was returned to the drinks cabinet and Robert returned to the garage. He removed the nails from Smokey's paws and laid the cat on his work bench. Rigor mortis had set in and it was difficult to find a box big enough to contain the cat's body. In desperation he finally had to break the cat's legs to get it to fit inside the cardboard box which was to be its coffin. Robert had tears streaming down his cheeks as he picked up his spade and carried the box containing Smokey's body outside. He dug a hole in the top right-hand corner of the garden and buried the box under the ground. It seemed ironic to him that all around there were dead flower heads as if several wreaths had been strewn on the floor for Smokey's benefit. Some minutes later the whisky bottle was removed from the cabinet again.

Chapter 22

Through dark doors

He arrived back at the hospital just before midday looking and feeling like death. The doctor was waiting for him and took him to a private room to express his concerns about his patient. 'I really do not want to release her,' he said. 'In my view she needs urgent psychiatric help.' Robert told the doctor about Ruth's father and their experience of mental hospitals. She was just recovering from months of suffering from severe depression. 'If she were to be committed to a psychiatric unit now I think it would finish her.' The doctor shook his head, 'I'm sorry he went on, but clearly your wife is a danger to herself and to the people around her. In her current mental state to release her from specialist medical care would be irresponsible and should anything happen I would be held accountable.'

'Then please,' begged Robert. 'Just let me take her home for the rest of the weekend. I'll get my son to help and we'll watch her 24/7, I promise. It'll give me a chance to prepare the way. I can talk to her and hopefully explain that she is not being sectioned, merely being admitted to hospital for the shortest possible time to help her get well.

The doctor thought for some time and then reluctantly agreed for Ruth to be allowed home until Monday morning. But he warned Robert that if anything else were to happen he needed to seek help quickly. 'Ask yourself one thing,' he said, 'how would you feel if she kills herself or someone else for that matter?'

The Grim Reaper

Robert drove Ruth home fully aware of the enormity of the task ahead. Once home, he sat her in front of the television and put on one of her favourite old film classics, 'A love affair to remember,' starring Deborah Kerr and Cary Grant. He was given three bottles of tablets by the doctor and read the instructions again to ensure he knew exactly when they had to be taken. 'I will stay awake all night,' he said to himself, 'and then tomorrow I'll explain why she has to go into hospital just for a little while.'

True to his word, Robert sat at Ruth's bedside for most of the night. In the early hours of the morning he needed to use the toilet and went to the bathroom. As he was zipping up his trousers he noticed a red marker pen on the floor under the sink. He bent down to pick it up and was suddenly aware that it had been used to mark out a shape on the tiles of the bathroom floor. Right next to the bath, the shape of a body had been clearly outlined in red ink. The bathroom almost looked like a crime scene when investigators have drawn around a corpse. Robert reached for a flannel and tried unsuccessfully to remove the ink from the tiled floor. Picking up the pen, he read the word 'permanent'. He returned to the bedroom to keep his silent vigil again. Ruth was sleeping peacefully.

He awoke still sitting in his chair. It was daylight and bright beams of sunlight were streaming into the bedroom through a narrow chink in the curtains. Ruth was not in their bed. Robert shot onto his feet and raced to the landing. The bathroom door was slightly ajar and he could see that the light was on. He pushed the door open and focused on a bath full of blood-red water. Ruth's head was propped up on the rim of the bath and her limp arms were draped along the sides. Both wrists were slit and blood was oozing into the water and onto the floor. Robert lifted his unconscious wife from what he thought at the time was her watery grave and gently laid her body on the floor. She fitted the shape drawn in red ink perfectly as if some invisible hand had traced a line around her seemingly lifeless body. He checked for a pulse in her neck and was relieved to find a very faint one. He wrapped towels tightly around her wrists to stem the flow of blood and raised her legs on top of a wicker basket normally used to store dirty laundry. Racing back to the bedroom he grabbed the phone and dialled for an ambulance. Returning to Ruth, he sat by her side elevating her legs still further. Tears were streaming down his face. He held the towels at her wrists with his hands hoping more pressure would reduce her blood loss and quietly he kept repeating to her that he loved her and would always love her no matter what.

Ruth spent three days in the local hospital on the accident and emergency ward and was then admitted to Claymore Hospital. Sean drove his car whilst Robert went with her in the ambulance. For the whole of the journey she could not be reconciled to her fate. She begged Robert to take her home. She pleaded with the nurses who came to collect her from the ambulance. She was dragged kicking and screaming in through the dark unwelcoming doors. It was all Robert could do not to tear her from their grasp and take her home. They followed her up onto the ward where the doctor in charge of Ruth's case advised Sean to take Robert home. Father and son could both hear Ruth calling for Robert to save her, pleading, begging not to be left. 'She'll settle more quickly,' he said, 'if you're not here.' Sean could see how distraught his father was and did as he was bid.

The Grim Reaper

They had been back at home for less than ten minutes when the hospital rang. Ruth, wearing only a flimsy negligee, had managed to escape from the ward and had run onto the road outside the hospital. She had been hit by a car which fortunately had not been moving at speed. Nevertheless, she had a nasty cut to her head but no serious injuries. The voice on the phone asked Robert not to go back to the hospital that day. He was told that Ruth had been sedated and would sleep for several hours. The voice assured him that Ruth was safe and asked if he could bring more bed wear for his wife and some comfortable casual clothes in the morning. 'If she should wake and is upset, you will make sure someone calls me?' Robert urged.

'Of course,' the voice replied, hanging up the receiver. The next day when they arrived at Ruth's bedside she was still heavily sedated. All Robert could do was sit by her side, holding the hand not attached to a drip, and pray.

The following day when Robert visited, although still sedated, Ruth was conscious and able to speak. Robert discovered why she had been involved in a road accident. She hesitantly explained what had happened. She overheard the doctor telling one of the nurses that he intended to have Ruth sectioned. The doctor was expecting a colleague to examine Ruth later that day to give the necessary second opinion required to make the section legal. Ruth had panicked and fled the ward. She was so anxious to escape before the section could be authorised that she hadn't bothered to dress or put shoes on. In her desperation to get away, she ran out onto the road without looking. The car had hit her before she knew it. She was taken back to the ward. Even drugged as she was, Ruth begged Robert to take her home. 'I saw what they did to my father,' she pleaded.

'Please Robert take me home, take me home please, please.' Robert tried to comfort her. 'I will not let them section you, I promise. That is not going to happen to you. I give you my word,' he said with absolute conviction. It was to be a promise he would be unable to keep, as he was soon to discover.

Chapter 23

A Plea for help

What Ruth witnessed with her father in Claymore Hospital, Robert was now to witness with his wife. On his next visit to the hospital, the doctor, as expected, asked him to consent to Ruth being sectioned. Robert refused. The doctor urged him to reconsider, saying that it was in Ruth's best interests. Robert reiterated equally as firmly that he was not going to give his consent and was even more adamant that he would never give his consent. Ruth was sectioned four days later. Robert discovered that the Mental Health Act provides for certain patients detained under section 2 or 3 of the Act not only to be sectioned but also to be subject to compulsory treatment provisions. He was also to discover that electro-convulsive therapy and naso-gastric feeding could be authorised if an SOAD (Second Opinion Authorised Doctor) agreed to the treatments recommended by the case doctor. Robert soon realised he was powerless. Ruth was at the mercy of a medical system which seemed to Robert to be both archaic and brutal. Everything he witnessed on his daily visits reminded him of Victorian lunatic asylums and he slept badly every night, if at all.

Less than a week after Ruth's incarceration in Claymore Hospital, the monthly Electrical Contractors Association magazine was posted through Robert's front door. On the front cover was a picture of the Grim Reaper. The choice of picture was clearly intended to draw attention to an article about contractors using substandard materials to save money in the current economic climate. The article stated that materials were being used which were so substandard that peoples' lives were being put at risk. The picture of the Grim Reaper reminded Robert of LLangar church and he made an appointment that day to see the Bishop of Crawley. The Bishop lived in a large house on the Royal Crescent, an exclusive area of Crawley with grand Georgian houses overlooking the River Stour. The housekeeper who in an uncanny way resembled the old lady they met at Rug Chapel, showed Robert into the library. The Bishop did not keep him waiting long. Robert spoke at length, sparing no details. The Bishop listened intently and when he finally spoke, his words were carefully and deliberately chosen. 'Exorcism and the belief in demonic possession have been part of the Catholic faith for hundreds of years. If we believe in God, we must also believe in the devil. Devils are powerful beings and can be extremely harmful to the unqualified. I will visit your wife to assess whether she has been taken over by an evil entity or spirit. But I will not attempt an exorcism myself. I have a colleague who is far more experienced in these matters than I. Should I feel your wife needs his help, I will contact him and we will do what we can. Now, I'm sorry to cut our meeting short but I have other pressing matters to attend to. Be assured I will visit your wife within the next few days, make my assessment and get back to you. Be of good faith, you are no longer alone.' He took Robert's hands and shook them firmly. 'See to your health,' he said 'and try and get some sleep. We will all need to be strong when and if the time comes for us to act.'

Robert was shown out by the housekeeper and began to walk back to town. There was a spring in his step and for the first time in days he had hope again. He was half way up one of the main streets leading back into town known as Castle Rise, a particularly steep hill with shops on either side, when he saw a man turn the corner at the top. The man started to head down the hill

The Grim Reaper

towards him. Robert stopped in his tracks. The man was the exact image of the Grim Reaper he had seen on Sean's DVD. A tall, thin man with a ghastly white sickly complexion and deep, sunken eyes- piercing eyes which now appeared to be looking straight at him. The gaunt figure was dressed all in black and wearing a dark hooded coat. It seemed to float rather than walk towards him. Robert could see the awful eyes staring out from under the hood and he felt as if his brain was being pierced for information. Robert averted his gaze and continued up the hill. Their paths crossed as they reached the entrance to the Victoria Hotel about three-quarters of the way up. Robert avoided any eye contact. At the top of the hill he could not resist turning around. The Grim Reaper had also turned around and was looking up at him. He had stopped exactly where their paths had crossed. Robert could not fail to notice his expression. He was smiling and nodding, but it was an evil smile, contemptuous and cold as ice. Robert found his newly acquired sense of hope and optimism draining away into abject despair.

Chapter 24

Sense of evil

The Bishop of Crawley visited Claymore Hospital three days later. He had telephoned to say that he wished to visit three of the seven wards. He would like to be shown Ash, Sycamore and Oak wards. Ruth was in Sycamore ward, but he had been non-specific in his reasons. Nursing staff were instructed to make sure their ward was as clean as possible and in so far as they were able to make patients quiet, calm and presentable. From early morning, things did not go to plan. The patients on Sycamore ward seemed agitated and were particularly difficult to dress and feed. The noise in the ward was five times the normal level with patients shouting, cursing the nursing staff, using expletive after expletive. As the Bishop's car drew up in the car park below, Ruth remained in her bed covering her ears with her hands. Mayhem and madness reigned and the horrified nursing staff seemed helpless to contain it.

A number of patients managed to climb up onto the windowsills. Tortured faces were pressed against the glass and they began to wail, like lost souls desperate to be saved. The Bishop could hear the clamour, sensed their misery and felt pity beyond belief. He prayed for help to ease their suffering. Looking up at the windows of the ward the Bishop could plainly see the faces of despair, the traumatised minds and struggled to tear his eyes away from theirs. He ventured no further, got back into his car and drove away. He'd seen enough. He contacted his colleague that afternoon. 'It's worse than I thought,' he told him.

The Grim Reaper

'As soon as I arrived I felt an overwhelming sense of evil. That awful building has been exposed to almost two hundred years of violence, madness and human misery. If the poor woman is as sensitive to spiritual matters as I believe, goodness only knows how she is surviving. One thing is certain, however, we cannot perform an exorcism there.'

'Is it possible for the husband to have her home over a weekend perhaps?' the priest on the other end of the line enquired.

'Possibly,' replied the bishop. 'But if we were to perform an exorcism and then return her to that terrible place in the most vulnerable of conditions, without our protection,' the bishop stopped in his tracks and after a moment's pause, he concluded, 'she would be the lamb to Satan's slaughter.'

'Well,' the priest continued, 'we need to assess how strong the possession is. The husband will have to arrange for her to be allowed out. It would be best if we could visit the home where these disturbing events took place. I can guarantee that the demon will show his hand. He is nothing if not conceited. You will need to warn the husband, the demon will do all in his power to deter us. Does the husband believe?' the priest asked.

'He didn't say so, but I believe he has been influenced by an aunt and uncle who were very devout. They have formed him and he is ready I feel to confirm his faith. He would die rather than abandon his wife.'

Less than a week later, on a day when Robert had arranged for Ruth to be allowed home, headlines regarding the Bishop were on the front page of every newspaper. 'Catholic priest killed in head-on car crash. Bishop of Crawley critically ill in intensive care. Robert was unaware of the newspaper headlines. He collected Ruth from the ward at 10am as agreed with the nursing staff. She had to be returned by 6pm. The Bishop stated a clear intention of calling at their home, with his colleague, arriving by mid-day at the latest. This was to be a preliminary visit to assess Ruth's condition and bless their home. Robert drove straight back to the house from the hospital and since their arrival, had been anxiously pacing up and down. Ruth was made comfortable in the lounge and was watching television. She was very sleepy and lethargic however, which Robert attributed to the medication she had been given shortly before leaving the hospital. Had she not been so heavily drugged, she would have quickly observed the strain he was under. Every few minutes and each time a car drove past, Robert would rush to the window, expecting to see two men of the cloth approaching his front door.

The day past pleasantly enough but there were no visitors. Robert served tea at 4.30pm and Ruth seemed to appreciate the change from hospital food. She ate surprisingly well and seemed more cheerful than she had been in months. Her improved mood was short lived. Robert found it difficult to persuade her back to the car. She did not want to leave her home. On the drive back to the hospital, she became more and more agitated. As Robert parked the car in the hospital car park, she was crying pitifully, begging him to take her home again. She refused to get out of the car and as the 6 o'clock deadline passed, Robert was forced to telephone the ward from his mobile phone and ask for assistance. He wept as he watched his wife being dragged back onto the ward by two disinterested orderlies, talking football and oblivious to the desperate pleas of the woman they had at their mercy. Robert sat for some time in his car before driving home. He stopped for petrol on route and it was then that he saw the headlines referring to the Bishop's accident. Robert was physically sick at the side of the car.

Chapter 25

Father and son

Sean found him the next morning. He had been ringing to find out how his mother's day at home had gone. He wanted to call round to see her, but Robert advised against it, saying that she would find it too much to bear. They should wait until there had been more of an improvement in her mental state. Sean had reluctantly agreed. When Sean opened the kitchen door he found Robert slumped over the dining table, with an empty whisky bottle standing like a witness for the prosecution at its centre. He put the kettle on and within minutes a mug of steaming black coffee had come to Robert's defence. Robert slowly gathered his wits and rallied his spirits sufficiently enough to be able to speak. 'I gather the day didn't go well,' Sean said, nodding at the empty whisky bottle protruding out of the waste bin. Robert tried to speak, but instead, tears rolled down his face and he covered his eyes with his hands. All he could do was to shake his head. Sean sprang to his feet and embraced his father. 'Come on old man,' he said compassionately, 'it's not like you to get so downhearted. We've all got to stay strong, for Mum's sake.'

'I know, I know,' Robert replied, finally managing to compose himself.

'Listen,' said Sean, 'and I'm not taking 'no' for an answer, once you've had a shower and some breakfast, you and I are going out for the day on our bikes.'

'No,' said Robert.' I'd love to of course, but I really must go and see that your mother is OK. She was distraught

The Grim Reaper

when I had to take her back yesterday,' and again the tears began to flow.

Sean spoke in his most authoritative voice, 'Dad, if you don't take some time out and start looking after yourself more, you're going to be ill as well. Where will that leave Mum then? I'm going to cook us some breakfast, whilst you take a shower and get ready and then hangover or not, we're going out for the day on our bikes.

A full English breakfast later, Robert was wheeling his bike out to join his son. 'Where are we going?' he asked

'It's a surprise,' replied Sean, pulling down his visor. 'Just follow me and try to stay up old man,' he goaded playfully. Sean decided on a route which connected the town of Welshpool with the Berwyn mountain range. They followed a route along the A490 and then pulled off to join the B4391. This road, not for the faint-hearted, would take them across the top of the Berwyn range. It was a breathtaking ride. After passing through a few scenic villages with great valley and mountain views, the road rose to snake across the mountains which ran along the boundary of the Snowdonia National Park. Robert began to feel life was almost worth living again as the bike sped around sweeping bends, dropped steeply into plummeting dips and clung to the side of distracting, sheer drops which illuminated the highland section of their route. Then they began a gradual descent through green farmland and dense woods and all the while, with a backdrop of spectacular pine forests and rugged mountains to admire.

They pulled off into a lay-by which had a roadside catering van. The bikes were propped up on their stands and father and son sat on the grass verge to enjoy a can of coke and a ham sandwich. Robert was about to bite into his, when he felt as if his mouth was being forced open by some invisible hand. He tried to speak, but could not move his tongue. He tried to move his arms but they felt pinned down and his eyes immediately focused on Sean with a look of blind terror. Sean, seeing that something was clearly wrong, rushed to Robert's side and to his horror watched his father's body suddenly jerk violently. Robert's back arched upwards as his whole body stiffened and shook. He made a loud guttural groan and then slowly his body returned to normal. There was blood on Roberts lip. 'Dad, Dad, are you OK?' Sean asked with a trembling voice.

Robert wiped the blood from his mouth with a shaking hand. 'Yes, I'm alright, just bitten my tongue,' he said. 'But I think your mother has had her first electric shock treatment!' Just as Robert identified the first time he had experienced a kind of mental telepathy with his wife, now he was to recognise the last time. From that day on, it was as if the psychic connection between them had been shattered, it would never happen again.

Chapter 26

To fight alone

Robert made constant enquiries as to the Bishop's health for several days and was relieved when it was announced that the Bishop was expected to make a full recovery. Finally, the Bishop returned home and Robert wasted no time arranging an appointment to see him. He rang the doorbell and stood for several minutes in a cold wind and driving rain before a stone -faced housekeeper eventually admitted him in to warm and welcoming hall. He was shown through to the library where the bishop, sitting in a wheelchair, had been reading. The Bishop looked up and seeing Robert being ushered in through the door, he closed his book and requested that the housekeeper bring them some tea.

It was a long and difficult conversation. The Bishop confirmed his heartfelt concern for Robert and Ruth and in particular his belief that demonic possession might well lie as the root cause of Ruth's ongoing problems and mental decline. He read from the Bible and Robert listened quietly to Luke 8 where Christ casts out demons from a man called Legion. The Bishop reiterated that exorcism the practice of casting out demons is an accepted and necessary practice of Roman Catholic faith, but he also pointed out the pitfalls. He did not feel that after his recent accident he was in a position to help whilst Ruth remained sectioned. 'I felt the strong presence of evil in that hospital,' he said. 'Until we remove her from that environment I would be concerned that we might do more harm than good and unleash powers beyond our control.'

Robert found himself nodding in agreement. 'I fully understand your concern, Bishop,' he replied ardently. 'I only hope that my asking you to help has not also put you at risk, bearing in mind your recent accident.'

'Do not think of me,' the Bishop replied vehemently. 'You must concentrate solely on your own affairs. Now listen carefully, this is of utmost importance. You must continue to pray, God has not abandoned you. You must fight for your wife to be released from her section. That's the key. Once she's home, once we can control her situation and protect her, then and only then can we act with safety and certainty that this demon can and will be driven out. I will pray for you and you, Mr Weston, must put your faith in Christ. Keep me informed and as soon as you have achieved your goal, the very moment your wife steps across your threshold once more and into your care, I will arrange for a priest to visit. Do not be down-hearted, that is what the demon wants. He will try to destroy your hope. He will try to make you weak in your resolve. You must stay strong and you will need your faith for that.'

Robert returned into the chill wind and driving rain. He walked slowly back to his car going over in his mind all that the Bishop had said. He would take his advice, he would pray, he would ask for God's help. But, he now knew for sure, that only he could help Ruth and until they had beaten the section order, the Church and the Bishop remained impotent and unable to help. He would have to fight the battle alone through the courts. Robert did not contact the Bishop again and felt that whilst their situation remained as it was, all hope from that quarter was lost.

The months passed and Robert continued his legal fight. He wrote to his local Member of Parliament to complain, detailing incidents and treatments he had seen first-hand what could only be described as torture, inhuman, degrading and at times more like a punishment. He hired solicitor after solicitor at great financial cost to fight the doctors and get her released from the section ruling, but it was all to no avail. He insisted on second opinions being sought and eventually achieved a breakthrough. The doctors at Claymore Hospital would not agree to the lifting of the section on Ruth, but they did agree that she could be transferred to another hospital. Robert made hundreds of enquiries until a clinic in London offered to take her. When he visited, the people he spoke to seemed so different to the Claymore hospital medical staff whose disinterest and lack of humanity he had come to expect. The London nurses were helpful, interested and concerned. Robert had no hesitation in accepting their offer and Ruth was transferred just before Christmas in 2008. Once again, Robert had reason to hope.

Chapter 27

Sledgehammer to crack a nut

It was a Sunday afternoon and Elizabeth was ironing as usual. It was her least favourite job, but it had to be done. Elizabeth always ironed to one of her favourite films, one she could listen to and visualise without needing to look up at the television screen. She was watching the final episode of the Poldark series. This was the one she enjoyed watching the most. The spectre of Elizabeth Warleggan no longer haunted the marriage of the two central characters and Demelza - the central female character - was telling Ross - the central male character, 'that you cannot fear death. Death is a certainty that we all face. All we can do is to live every day to the full. All we will ever have is the here and the now.' Elizabeth noticed a movement at the window and looked up. A fat, well fed squirrel was hanging upside down from the bird table outside and gnawing at the seed ball suspended below it. There was a loud knock at the door, and the squirrel dropped to the ground and raced off.

Elizabeth went to open the door and standing in the hallway she found her much changed brother. His once dark hair was now completely grey and worry lines were etched around his eyes and across his forehead. He looked old, tired and beaten. 'Robert, my God!' she exclaimed. 'Come in, come in. How are you, we haven't seen you in months, years?' Robert made a few polite enquiries into Elizabeth's family situation and then explained that he had come with something particular to say.

The Grim Reaper

'I want to apologise for not coming to see you for so long and not keeping touch.' Elizabeth was relieved, for some time now she had been convinced she had somehow offended him. Every time she had invited his family over for a meal or to stay during holiday times, which they had always done in the past, the invitation was declined. Robert began his account.

Elizabeth listened in silence. 'She's lost a lot of teeth due to the electro shock therapy. They put a rubber device in your mouth to prevent you from biting your tongue or breaking your teeth, but when you're fighting against the treatment, sometimes they make mistakes. I've done a huge amount of research into the procedure and all the recommendations are that it is just a quick fix. It pacifies the patient in the short term, but does nothing to address the underlying problems, which re-surface once the effects have worn off. They do it to raise the level of a substance called,' he paused for a moment, 'called serotonin I think. It's a substance which acts as an inhibitory brain chemical. What it does is enhance repression and renders the person devoid, bereft of emotional memory for days, weeks and sometimes forever. The treatment is monstrous Lizzie and so unnecessary. What they've done to Ruth is criminal. Many patients are dying every year in NHS psychiatric hospitals due to the dangerous combinations of psychotropic drug treatment they're given. The treatment is often enforced against both the patient's and their relatives' wishes. That's the problem you see, the doctors can do what they like when the patient is under section. Over a million NHS patients in the UK are currently addicted to prescribed psychotropic drugs.'

'Over a million, I can't believe it!' Lizzie exclaimed, 'I had no idea this problem even existed let alone how many people were affected. That's awful, Robert, really awful!'

'Worse still, Robert continued, 'hundreds of thousands have suffered brain and other damage due to the side effects of these toxic drug treatments. The damage is in many cases irreversible and therefore untreatable. So many doctors have concluded that antidepressant treatment is like using a sledgehammer to crack a nut, especially in cases of mild to moderate depression. Bombarding a delicate person with external and often toxic chemicals on a long-term basis is bound to create unpleasant side effects. In Ruth's case, side effects from which she will never now recover. You wouldn't recognise her Lizzie, she so damaged. It's pitiful to see the way she is. What they have done is wicked, really wicked. She cannot bear to look at herself in a mirror.' Robert went on to say that his only objective in life now was to get Ruth home. 'I know I'll never be able to make her well again Lizzie, the best I can hope for is to stop her suffering.

There's something else Lizzie, something I want you to know, but I'm afraid of frightening you!'

'What is it?' she asked.

Robert told her about their experiences and their belief that they had been and were still, albeit to a lesser extent, being subjected to the malice of an evil entity. 'It sounds madness I know to say, but it is as if the Grim Reaper has haunted our existence since the death of Ruth's mother and especially since our visit to Llangar church. Something happened to Ruth in that church Lizzie, something terrifying and sinister. There have been so many other things Lizzie, so many events that have happened which have no logical explanation. Each time something happens I try to account for it, to make

The Grim Reaper

myself believe that perhaps I just imagined it, but in my heart of hearts I know our lives have been overshadowed by this demon. It's true Lizzie, what they say. There are more things in heaven and earth!'

When he left, Elizabeth stood in the doorway watching his car disappear down the drive. She had the awful feeling that he had come to say a final goodbye and an equally awful conviction that everything he had said was absolutely true. She shivered as a chill swept through her body.

Chapter 28

A ray of hope

Robert felt he had scored a victory. The doctor at Claymore Hospital agreed that Robert could transport Ruth to the new clinic in London in his own car. He booked a double room in a hotel not far from the clinic and decided to spend a peaceful night alone with his wife before admitting her to the clinic. He parked the car in the hotel car park, checked in and received his room keys. Ruth was all too aware of her appearance and so Robert had been charged with finding a back way into the hotel, avoiding the need to walk through a crowded reception area. He had done just that and now at last after such a long time apart, they were finally alone in the privacy of their own room if not their own home. The room had its own en-suite bathroom and Robert immediately ran a bath for Ruth adding in some of her favourite lavender oil. She was very shaky on her feet and her trembling fingers struggled to undo her buttons. Robert sat by her on the side of the bed and helped her to undress. He had not seen her naked for some considerable time. He helped her to her feet and guided her into the bathroom. The bath looked warm and inviting and Ruth smiled up lovingly at him as he helped her to lie down in the comforting water. He gently washed her hair.

'Do I disgust you now?' Ruth suddenly said with a voice tinged with sadness. 'Skin and bone, that's all I am nowadays,' she continued.

'Neither of us have the figures we once had,' Robert replied, 'nor does everything I have seem to have dropped. Although some of it has- you'll forgive me if I'm not specific.'

The Grim Reaper

'When I come home, we'll go climbing and walking again like we used to,' she said more cheerfully.

'You bet we will,' he agreed, kissing her gently on the forehead. 'You have a good soak and I'll make us some tea.' Leaving the bathroom Robert returned to the bedroom and switched on the kettle. He sank on to the bed and covered his eyes with his hands. The sight of Ruth's decrepit, withered body had shocked him. The kettle boiled and Robert made the tea, blinking away the tears which insisted on welling up in his eyes. 'If our eyes are the windows to our soul,' he thought to himself, 'I need mine to look bright and normal, not red and swollen. I must pull myself together for Ruth's sake.'

The next morning they left for the clinic. They were greeted by Ruth's new doctor and escorted up to the ward. Ruth was to have a private room, however, and Robert helped unpack her clothes and night attire into a small locker to one side of her bed. The room had a window overlooking a garden of lawn and herbaceous borders. Stone paths criss-crossed the garden, lined with wooden benches and picnic tables. Robert once more felt they had a real chance of overcoming Ruth's illness and getting her home. Hope returned and his spirits were lifted. The doctor explained that Ruth would now undergo a series of tests. 'Having read your notes,' he said, 'I wonder if your initial problems might have been caused by diabetes. Anyway, we'll do our best for you,' he said reassuringly 'and investigate ways in which your medication could slowly be reduced. It will take time however, but we will try to make you as comfortable as we can while you're here.' Both Robert and Ruth thought they had died and gone to heaven. In the afternoon they were able to take advantage of the warm weather and enjoyed a short stroll together in the garden. Robert was allowed to stay until well after supper time and it was just after 10pm when he finally kissed his wife goodnight and made his way back down to the ground floor.

Robert noticed there was a small room acting as a chapel, just to the right of the reception desk. He had not been to church for some time and he decided before driving back to the hotel that he ought to express his thanks to God. Since his last meeting with the Bishop of Crawley he had been so busy with his legal battles to get Ruth released from her section that he had little time to pray. However, since his meeting with the staff at the London clinic he felt such high hopes for Ruth's recovery that he wanted to let God know. He wanted to pray and tell God that at last things were moving in the right direction and that help from above would always be appreciated.

The chapel was quite deserted. It was pleasantly decorated. The oak floor had a central floral carpet and an altar at the front was decorated with vases of white daises at each end and had a golden cross and leather bound Bible at its centre. The room was lined with beige upholstered chairs and mahogany-coloured silk curtains framed tall windows which stretched the length of two entire walls. There was a confessional box in one corner of the room and although not Roman Catholic himself, Robert found himself entering and sitting down.

He had always been a private sort of person and the confessional box would afford him privacy from any spying eyes. He sat down and began to talk quietly to himself, expressing his sadness for all the traumatic experiences he and Ruth suffered over the years, but his hope now for a better future. As he prayed he was suddenly aware of how cold he had become. The air temperature had inexplicably dropped and as he prayed his breath was turning into an icy vapour. He felt a chill

The Grim Reaper

run through his body. It was then that he realised he was no longer alone in the confessional. A face could be seen on the opposite side of the grille. At first, he thought he had been joined by a priest coming to take his confession. Then, very slowly, he recognised the black hood, the sunken hollow eyes and the white, sickly complexion and froze to his core as he watched a black toothless mouth curve into a monstrous, evil smile. The mouth seemed to be rasping for breath as if about to speak. Robert tore out of the confessional box, ripping the velvet curtain from its rail as he did so. He ran back up to the ward, insisting the staff check on Ruth again. It took some time for the night nurse to reassure him all was well. Finally, and by now feeling exhausted, he returned to the hotel.

Robert entered their hotel room and bolted the door behind him. His heart was racing and he could not even consider going to bed. He tidied up the room and drank coffee after coffee, willing the hours by so that he could return to the hospital and check that Ruth had come safely through the night. He could not stop from trembling. The sight of the Grim Reaper in the confessional box horrified him and he was filled with dread. As the night wore on and the caffeine took effect, he began to wonder whether had simply imagined seeing that awful presence again. He knew he'd been on a roller coaster of emotions over recent days. The relief he felt driving Ruth away from Claymore Hospital, knowing she need never return. The joy at spending a night together albeit tinged with a terrible sadness at how her poor body had aged during her long years of confinement. The elation of seeing her settle into her private room in the new clinic and for the first time in so many months surrounded by nursing staff who seemed to care. He knew he had been deprived of sleep for months and over the past three nights he had not slept at all. As morning light dawned, he tried to convince himself that what he experienced the night before was all in his imagination, an imagination which he believed had been driven by fatigue and anxiety. He could not bear the thought that Ruth could still be at the mercy of the Grim Reaper.

Chapter 29

Permanent damage

On the first night Ruth arrived at the clinic in London she suffered an unexpected brain seizure and was discovered not breathing by a nurse on early morning duty. She was put on a ventilator and it was touch and go for several days as to whether or not she would survive. Robert stayed by her side, praying all the while that the Grim Reaper would not take her from him. He wished he had stayed with her throughout that first night. He believed the visitation of the Reaper in the confessional box had been a warning. It was a warning he should have heeded and he was filled with regret that he had not stayed to protect her. Ruth choked on her own vomit during the seizure and there was real concern that being starved of oxygen, she may have suffered brain damage as a result. Robert prayed throughout his waking hours for her to be well.

Much to his relief, Robert's prayers were finally answered and slowly Ruth began to recover. Various tests were carried out which showed the sodium levels in her body from the drugs she was given were too low. Ruth had been taking a lithium medication which depletes sodium levels in the body for a considerable time and it was thought this may have caused the brain seizure.

Ruth's condition was now worse. The only saving grace was that conditions at the clinic were considerably better that they had been at Claymore. Ruth had her own private room and Robert noticed that she seemed much more comfortable and relaxed than she had been in months. Treatment was by consent only and so the frightening, painful electro shock therapies ceased. However, Ruth had developed certain mannerisms she could not control. She had a habit of jutting her tongue out every few seconds and experienced sudden and violent twitches in her limbs. Robert asked to see a specialist who confirmed she had cerebral trauma, a condition which could not be cured. He also confirmed this condition could have been caused by the treatment she received and that any improvement to be expected would be minimal. Robert and Ruth had learned their lesson. They did not complain, they accepted their lot and waited patiently. 'We mustn't rock the boat!' Robert would say to Ruth. 'Have faith, stay strong, we will get you out of here.'

After months of Robert driving to and fro between Crawley and London, Ruth was released from her section and went home with Robert. She had served her long and cruel internment but Robert was about to begin his. Ruth needed constant attention and they found themselves unable to reduce her drug intake. Any doctor Robert contacted to help in this matter declined. Robert believed because he had challenged the medical profession on their treatment of Ruth specifically and the mentally ill in general, he had now been blacklisted. No one was prepared to help. It was as if they all closed ranks. Ruth also had to have a special diet. She lost so many of her teeth during her time in hospital and found chewing difficult. Most of her food had to be specially prepared and then mashed. Meal times were not pleasurable anymore and Robert found it painful to watch Ruth struggle to eat, in spite of the fact that she always put on a brave face.

Chapter 30

Final decisions

She was unable to see her grandchildren because they found her appearance and mannerisms frightening. Time and again family reunions failed and the children had to be taken away. On such occasions, Robert would remind Ruth how much better off they were than when she incarcerated in that awful hospital. Ruth would agree and say sadly 'There was nothing to like about that hateful place. I felt as if I were in hell. Having the freedom to leave and the knowledge I don't need to go back is everything. And most of all,' she would add, 'just to be with you again I could not wish for more.' Ruth had been at home for over a year but there was little, if any, improvement in her condition. They tried once more to make the grandchildren accept her, but they could not. Freya, in particular, had been truly frightened by her grandmother's appearance. The planned family dinner had been abandoned and Ruth and Robert were left sitting alone in their kitchen. 'I'm tired,' said Ruth.

'I know,' replied Robert. An air of despair hung over the kitchen like a blanket of autumn fog. Ruth's protruding tongue and its unwanted protrusion was the only predictable thing in their lives. 'I sometimes feel as if the Grim Reaper has won,' said Robert, 'he's virtually destroyed our lives.'

'We can beat him,' said Ruth with conviction. 'He wants to hurt us now. This is Hell, this is where it exists, on Earth,' she said. 'I've been on the brink of death so many times but he has always brought me back to suffer more.'

'But can you ever forgive me?' Robert asked as tears welled in his eyes. 'I feel I have brought all this suffering on us, through my own stupid vanity and selfish pride. I should have asked for help long ago, instead of acting like the proverbial ostrich and sticking my head in the sand, hoping that your illness would just go away. Everyone thought we had the perfect marriage. I couldn't bring myself to let anyone see the slightest blemish. I deliberately hid your illness from everyone, even our son. It was wrong and shameful of me. I've brought you to this, how can you ever forgive me?'

'Robert, you must not think like that. How do you know that if you had asked for help earlier, I would not have been sectioned earlier? At the beginning of my illness the doctors would still have bombarded my body with all kinds of toxic chemicals. I would still have looked like this and been like this, possibly years earlier. Your stubbornness not to admit we had an insurmountable problem, your determination to protect me, has prolonged our time together and delayed my suffering. I truly believe you were sent to be my knight in shining armour, to stave off for as long as possible the misery that was to come. '

'But, it's criminal, inhuman and wicked,' Robert sobbed, 'what they have done to you.'

'And yet you still love me, as much now as on the day we were married,' she said. 'How many men would stay loyal and loving towards their wives with all that we have had to face? My darling, I have nothing to forgive. You are my rock, my foundation and my heart is and always will be yours. Robert dried his eyes and pulled her to him, cradling her in his arms. 'Do you believe Robert?' she said, 'I mean really believe?'

'How can I not?' he replied, taking her hand in his.

The Grim Reaper

'We were too happy,' she said, 'we drew his attention.' Robert nodded and kissed her forehead tenderly.

'My one, my only love,' he said embracing her tenderly.

Their decision was made. It only remained to spend a special day with Sean. Robert rang Sean that evening. 'Are you working on Friday?' he asked.

'No, I'm not as it happens, Dad. Why, what have you got in mind?'

'Another great day out on our bikes whilst this good weather lasts and to pacify Vicky, how would she like it if I take her and the girls to the cinema on Saturday, whilst you spend the day catching up with your mother?'

'Sound's great Dad, I'll speak to Vicky and phone you back. Less than ten minutes later all arrangements had been made.

Chapter 31

Robert's goodbye

Sean arrived on his motorbike at 10am sharp. The family sat in the kitchen chatting over a cup of coffee. Robert and Sean kissed Ruth goodbye and set off on their bikes. 'Where are we going?' Sean asked.

'It's a surprise,' Robert replied, echoing a conversation of the not too distant past between father and son. 'Just follow me and try to stay up with the maestro, Junior,' Robert said with a wide grin. They reached Bala at midday and stopped for an early lunch. 'Your mother and I love this place, Robert said.

'I can see why,' replied Sean, admiring the scenery. The vast expanse of water sparkled in the bright sunshine and fields of green and a clear blue sky served only to enhance the view.

'Now,' said Robert, 'you're going to enjoy this route, but beware. There are two really sharp bends as the road climbs out of Bala and a few miles off, the mother of all hairpins! Keep your bike under control, you know the score.'

'I know, I know, Sean replied, 'speed and safety, hand in hand, know your limits, need I go on?'

Robert laughed. 'Well at least something I've said has actually gone in!' It was a glorious route and both father and son were in their element. Robert led and Sean decided to let him own the day, staying a good twenty yards back throughout the ride. At Llyn Trawsfynydd they parked their bikes and sat outside a little coffee shop which had a number of tables and chairs set out on a small patio area which boasted full views of the lake. It felt good to relax and to enjoy the warmth of the early autumnal sunshine on their backs.

'What's the prognosis on Mum?' Sean asked during an unaccustomed break in the conversation.

Robert took a few minutes before replying. 'Not good,' he said. The cerebral trauma is irreversible. We've asked for a specialist in the field of neurology to assess the damage. The trouble is they would have to admit that the medical treatment she received caused her current condition and to get any branch of the medical profession to point the finger of blame in a specific direction is nigh on impossible. The various departments have all closed their doors and they all refuse to help us. No one will take our case on, so we've come to a dead end. They've closed ranks and so your mother is doomed to the life she now has now, self-imposed isolation, misery and suffering. A few years ago she asked me to help her end her life. We looked at those special clinics in Switzerland which advertise death with dignity.'

Before he could finish Sean interrupted, 'You can't consider that, Dad. I know you. It would kill you. You'd never be able to live with the guilt.'

'I know, said Robert, 'but can you understand how she feels? It's not just her own granddaughters who are afraid of how she looks, it's everyone. When she first came home I tried taking her out, but it was torture for her. Everywhere we went people would stare and make it clear from the expressions on their faces and their whispered conversations that we were unwelcome in their midst.

I remember once before you were born, taking her to a Little Chef Restaurant for a late breakfast when we going up to the lakes for a weekend. First time I took her over Hard Knott and Wrynose pass actually. There was this guy in the restaurant that clearly had Tourette's syndrome. He was sitting on his own at one of the tables and as soon as we sat down, I realised why everyone else in the restaurant was sitting as far from his table as possible. He kept calling out loudly and swearing about the poor service. He was expressing what we were all feeling. It took over three-quarters of an hour for our breakfast to come. Anyway, you know your mother, she had to go over to comfort him. 'Don't worry,' she said, 'your breakfast will be sorted as soon as they can manage. We're waiting for ours too. I think they're short-staffed today.' The Tourette sufferer smiled and as she walked back to our table, he said, 'What the fuck does she know!'

'What did mum do?' Sean asked.

'She just laughed,' Robert replied and said, 'Ah well at least I tried.' After a short pause, Robert continued, 'Anyway, your mother and I have been considering going away. Finding somewhere peaceful, quiet, where we can walk hand in hand and avoid the prying eyes of judgemental people.' Robert spoke gently, noting a fleeting expression of pain pass across Sean's face.

'People don't understand Dad, that's the trouble. They don't see the beautiful person Mum really is.'

'No they don't son and worse still, they never will. And the only way they are ever likely to is if they experience something similar themselves and I wouldn't wish that on my worst enemy.'

The Grim Reaper

'Well,' said Sean after several minutes of thoughtful silence, 'if you think going away will give you a better quality of life, of course I will support you every step of the way.'

'I knew you would understand,' Robert said tenderly. 'You know how proud we are of you, don't you? Your mother and I have watched you grow into a man with wonderful qualities. You have integrity, you're honest, hardworking and a loving and affectionate husband and father. We could not have wished for more. Just keep doing what you're doing. Whatever befalls you; know your strength, your courage, your ability to overcome whatever obstacle life may throw your way. You are your parent's son and we have done our best to arm you with a resilience no hardship can ever destroy. Live your life, take whatever it has to offer and above all, love. Love is everything. No father ever had a better son.' It was dark before they arrived back at Sean's house. Robert confirmed he would pick Vicky and the girls up at midday and Sean would spend the afternoon with his mother.

Chapter 32

Ruth's goodbye

When Sean arrived, Ruth was looking through old photo albums. They sat in the lounge together reminiscing about times gone by. When Robert and Ruth had married they had rented a small terraced cottage in the village of Stokesley. It was an ideal location being so close to the village of Kildale, where Keith built his bungalow. Almost every weekday from the age of three until he stared school Ruth took Sean to Stokesley Hall to explore the gardens. Sean had a little red and yellow three-wheeler trike. Ruth would attach a skipping rope to the handle bars to help pull him up the steep hills and control his speed on the fast downhill sections. She would often pack a picnic and they'd sit overlooking one of the many lakes on different levels that the gardens have to offer. Indeed the lakes comprise a veritable daisy- chain of water, beautifully planted with all manner of plants offering a colourful display of leaf and petal throughout the seasons. The lakes were also packed with fish, rainbow trout in particular as well as providing a rich habitat for a wide variety of ducks, moor hens, kingfishers and an exquisite pair of black swans. Sean would insist on taking some bread to feed the ducks on every visit. The fish, however, had other ideas, and Ruth would laugh at Sean's often vain attempts to make sure a particular duck got his fair share, when the fish would feast as furiously as they did. Often the water would look as if it was boiling. Fish would leap up out of the water and the floating bread would be gone in an instant.

The garden boasted an old donkey called Shamrock. Shamrock's stable and paddock was situated just outside the old walled garden. Every day Sean would take an apple or a carrot or some mints with which to feed the donkey. Shamrock grew to love Sean and Sean equally soon grew to love Shamrock. As time went by, it was clear that Shamrock recognised the sound of the three-wheeler trike approaching noisily on the tarmac roads which wound around the house and gardens. Shamrock would start to bray with all his might until his treat had duly been served.

Sean and Ruth slowly turned the pages of the albums. 'I remember that,' Sean repeated time and time again as he gazed at treasured photos. 'I can't think why I haven't taken Vicky and the girls there yet. You know, what I remember most about living at Stokesley were the seasons. I think Vicky would like to live somewhere warm all year round but I love England with its changing seasons. I am positive that I have you, dear mother and Stokesley Hall to thank for that.' They reminisced about how in the autumn they would walk through the woods admiring the changing colours of the leaves, leaves which now displayed their glorious kaleidoscope of autumn colours of brilliant reds, bright yellows and gleaming gold. They would often stand still and watch the wind slowly stripping the branches bare. Sean loved the sound of leaves rustling at his feet.

They loved the winter too, with its bright red holly berries and frost-encrusted cobwebs which hung in the hedgerow and were draped across every plant like diamond necklaces, sparkling in the sunshine. They would walk in warm coats, woollen hats, scarves, gloves and Wellington boots through snow-covered fields, testing the frozen ice between the stepping stones which criss-crossed the valley streams. Spring would follow winter and bring its masses of spring bulbs to life, the snowdrop, crocus, tulip, daffodils and all manner of tree blossom. The vast array of rhododendrons and camellias would herald early summer calling the azaleas, laburnums and lilacs into bloom.

Perhaps it was the summer that Sean and Ruth loved best, dressed now only in shorts, t-shirts and sandals, admiring the summer borders and their masses of hydrangeas, gladioli, geraniums, fuchsia and dahlia. In the summer the rose garden with its heady scent was their favourite port of call. At its centre, in a circle of lawn stood a large granite boulder on which Ruth had taught Sean the points of the compass. Sean was allowed to make a magic wish when he climbed to the top. His wish would only come true if he jumped down from the correct compass point. Ruth would call out North- for example- and Sean would make his choice and jump from the magic rock. Ruth would always cheer loudly as Sean made the correct choice and beamed a satisfied smile.

Most visits ended in the tea room. The tea room was the old trophy room. The passion of the 19th century aristocrat to hunt in far off foreign places was fully in evidence. The mounted heads of various wild beasts regaled every wall from floor to ceiling. African shields and spears guarded each door way. There were ancient glass cabinets full of stuffed birds from pelicans to parrots as well as cabinets full of snakes from puff adder to python. A taxidermist's skills were also on hand, with a fully grown stuffed lion and a Bengal tiger guarding the steps to the upper floor of the restaurant and each with bullet holes in its skin. Sean could press his fascinated fingers carefully into each hole. There were real teeth in a mouth you could safely put your hand in and just next door an ice cream cabinet containing your favourite lollipop. Sean's seeking eyes were never disappointed. The coffee shop was a treasure trove of mystery and adventure. At night time, Sean would chose an animal and Ruth would have to find a story to fit the bill.

Sean remembered everything about Stokesley and decided that would be his next destination on a family trip out with Vicky and the girls. 'I doubt old Shamrock will still be there though.'

'Will you take the girls' bikes?' Ruth asked laughing.

'Of course,' Sean replied 'it's a family tradition.'

'Do you know,' Ruth said smiling, 'it wouldn't surprise me if I found out that you or your dad invented the wheel in a past life. It wouldn't surprise me at all.' It was a wonderful day and unlike losing her father, she left Sean in no doubt as to how much she loved him. Mother and son enjoyed a long, warm embrace before he finally departed.

Chapter 33

Stairway to heaven

The trip this time was in the reverse order. They visited Llangar Church first and laid a dozen white tulips at the door as a sign of forgiveness, but they did not go in. At Rug Chapel they said prayers kneeling before the altar. It was midday when they reached Lake Bala, the sun was shining and the air was warm. Robert laid a picnic out on a blanket on an elevated grassy bank overlooking the lake. Ruth lay back in the sunshine looking up at the sky. 'We need to make the most of this walk,' she said.

'We will my darling,' he replied, 'we will.' They walked hand in hand around the lake, watching the birds and the wildlife and the water sport enthusiasts making the most of the fine weather. Slowly a red sun began to set behind the now dark mountains and the light was fading as they made their way back to the car. Gradually people were leaving, packing up their picnics, mooring their boats, lashing windsurfers to racks on the top of cars. Finally there was silence and night had fallen. The lake was deserted, only Robert and Ruth remained to keep it company.

'You know,' Ruth said, 'even after all that we have had to endure, I feel that God has blessed us, truly blessed us. How many people have known a love like ours? We are lucky Robert, to have experienced a love so deep, so passionate and yet so tender. An ever-fixed mark, that has looked on tempests but has never been shaken,' she said, quoting her favourite sonnet, the words of which seemed to her to encapsulate the essence of their marriage with all the struggles they had been forced to overcome.

'I've loved you from the first,' Robert replied, pulling her slender and tired body to him and holding her close, 'and I shall love you to the last.'

Robert drove the car up to the water's edge. He left the engine running, the music playing and the car doors open. They walked hand in hand across the pebbles on the shoreline. The silver, melancholy rays of a crescent moon silhouetted the outlines of their comparatively small frames against the vast expanse of water which stretched in front of them and graced their steps with light. Gentle waves lapped once more at their feet, their knees, their waists, their necks and then over their heads. The melancholic strains of 'Stairway to Heaven,' followed them into the water.

'There's a feeling I get,

When I look to the west,

And my spirit is crying,

For leaving

Their hands remained tightly gripped even in death.

Sean found the letter addressed to him on their mantel shelf later that day. The last lines read, 'We will rest in peace now, together. Be happy for us son, always strive to be happy and forgive us. We will always love you.'

Chapter 34

Sean's Inheritance

It was raining heavily and the rest of the mourners had returned to their cars and set off for the wake. Only Sean and Elizabeth remained at the grave side. 'Are you going to be OK?' she said anxiously.

'I have to be,' he replied wearily. 'I just wish there was something I could do to put things right. Dad felt so strongly about what happened to Mum. I think it broke him when he realised he was powerless to help in Mum's unfolding tragedy. We went on a bike ride you know, just before.' His voice faltered and in his emotion he could not speak. Lizzie put her arm around his waist. When he composed himself, he continued. 'It cost them dear both in terms of health and finance. Paying for all those solicitors took almost all their savings! When I think of the treatment Granddad and Mum received it makes me so angry. It really was appalling. Can you not see Aunt Lizzie how abysmal the standard of NHS mental health treatment and care is in the UK? Dad used to say that the situation was made far worse by the absolute legal powers of enforcement and removal of all human rights contained within mental health legislation. He tried so hard Aunt Lizzie, he tried so hard to get help.'

'I know,' she replied, 'don't upset yourself like this.'

'But I feel I need to fight his battle now. It's too late for Mum and Dad, but just maybe if people know what happened to them, some other poor soul won't have to suffer as they did.'

The Grim Reaper

'Come on,' Aunt Lizzie said as the rain began to fall even harder. 'Your wife and those two lovely girls need you now, more than ever.'

A torrent of water was by this time running down the steep path leading up to the main gate of the cemetery. Sheltering under Sean's large umbrella they slowly made their way through the grave stones. Wet feet trudged a sombre path, until Sean once again unburdened his dark thoughts on his aunt.

'The worst thing for Dad was that he found a total lack of any effective rights of appeal and was convinced that the various regulatory authorities have for years found it easier to simply turn a blind eye to what is going on, rather than do something about it. You know, he actually said to me that he could understand how Harold Shipman got away with killing so many patients over so many years without any action being taken. That last day we had together, he said his biggest regret was his failure to get the truth recognised. His overriding hope was that the truth about all this NHS abuse not only of mental health care but also elderly patients gradually emerges into the public domain. He believed increased public awareness would eventually lead to improved legislation. The legislation is the key, Aunt Lizzie. If legislation could be improved, it would result in giving better protection to patients and provide a better route to legal action through the courts in cases of abuse or medical mistakes.'

'He said as much to me when he came to visit me all those months ago,' his Aunt Lizzie recalled sadly, 'and you know I think he was right in what he believed, in that it is the only way to ensure NHS standards of care are improved.'

They reached the car. Sean held the umbrella over his aunt whilst she climbed inside and sat on the front passenger seat. Moments later, Sean turned the ignition key, switched on the wipers and glanced across at his aunt. She looked soaked to the skin and dark tracks of black mascara traced a mixed path of raindrops and tears down the flushed cheeks of her face.

'You read that sonnet beautifully in the service,' she said, aware that his eyes were on her.

'I read it for mum,' he replied with real tenderness in his voice. His aunt was reminded of just how much she loved him.

'We have to be happy and optimistic now, for both their sakes,' she said.

'I'm going to strive to be happy and if I can be half the man my father was, I'll truly be happy,' Sean said proudly.

'Aunt Lizzie, how would you like to come to Stokesley Hall with Vicky and me and the girls next Sunday?' Sean enquired as the car pulled away from the cemetery gates.

'I'd love to,' she replied. 'The last time I was there was with your father and your Great Aunt Mary and Uncle Jack. The house is Victorian you know and was used as a hospital for wounded soldiers during World War II. Your Great Aunt worked as a nurse there and she loved the place. There are beautiful lakes to walk around and the gardens are quite delightful.'

'I know,' he replied, 'you're forgetting I practically lived there as a small boy.'

The Grim Reaper

'Oh yes,' she said remembering. 'How remiss of me to forget those happier times, but, are you sure the memories won't be too raw?'

'Perhaps,' he replied, 'but they were really wonderful years. I loved that old cottage and Mum and I spent hours at the Hall. We visited the gardens almost every day. I'd like to remember her there, laughing at me trying to feed the ducks and playing hide-and-seek in the woods.' Sean suddenly stopped the car, overcome with emotion. It was some time before he could speak. Finally he turned to his aunt and with a voice thick with grief, he said, 'we'll get their message out, won't we Aunt Lizzie?'

'Damn right we will,' she replied, 'even if we have to shout their story from the rooftops, and we'll keep on shouting until somebody listens!'

The rain hammered down on the roof of the car. Rivulets of water streamed down the windows washing away the grime and the dirt until at last a break in the clouds allowed a beam of sunlight to penetrate an otherwise grey sky and the rain stopped. A God spot opened up and bright yellow rays from a small patch of blue sky seemed to target the stationary car and its two melancholy passengers sitting quietly below. Sunlight gathered about them and the whole interior of the car was suddenly illuminated with a golden glow. The rain, the tears would dry. The pain and grief would ease with time, but the love and the memory of a loved one's suffering would remain for all eternity.

Lightning Source UK Ltd.
Milton Keynes UK
24 March 2011

169756UK00001B/10/P